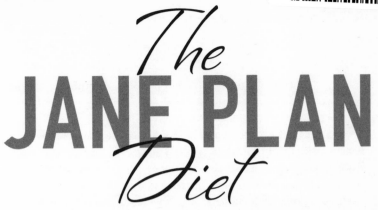

The JANE PLAN Diet

Life-changing weight loss from the woman who knows

JANE MICHELL

with Jane Garton

pıatkus

PIATKUS

First published in Great Britain in 2014 by Piatkus

A CIP catalogue record for this book
is available from the British Library.

ISBN 978-0-349-40353-3

Designed and typeset in Albertina and Vista Sans by Paul Saunders
Printed and bound in Great Britain by Clays Ltd, St Ives plc

Papers used by Piatkus are from well-managed forests
and other responsible sources.

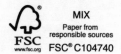

MIX
Paper from
responsible sources
FSC
www.fsc.org   FSC® C104740

PIATKUS
An imprint of
Little, Brown Book Group
100 Victoria Embankment
London EC4Y 0DY

An Hachette UK Company
www.hachette.co.uk

www.piatkus.co.uk

For everyone out there who is fed up
with diet fads and wants an easy approach to
a healthier, happier weight

CONTENTS

ACKNOWLEDGEMENTS

I WOULD LIKE TO THANK my long-suffering family who, since the beginning of the 'Jane Plan' journey, have put up with my many absences. My amazing children, William, Olivia and Tom: your endless encouragement, support and understanding about all things Jane Plan have made this book possible. When the going gets tough I think of you. In particular, my gorgeous daughter Olivia, who has recipe-tested, tasted and created, deserves a special mention. Olivia, you're always there with a positive smile and a practical approach – I am a truly lucky mother. I couldn't have done any of it without you.

From my team, the biggest thanks goes to Jane Garton for her patience, understanding of and belief in all things Jane Plan. Your skill with a pen has made this book readable and fun! Thank you Jane for your unending commitment.

Thanks to the fabulous girls at Jane Plan HQ: Kirsty Corcoran, Alexandra Dabrowska, Rachel Hunter and the rest of the team – your love of the work we do at Jane Plan makes every day a pleasure.

Thank you to my agent Heather Holden-Brown for her persistence and belief in Jane Plan, to Anne Lawrance for taking me on and to Jillian Stewart for her brilliant editing skills. Anna Cowie deserves a special mention for her inspirational illustrations and designs, and Laurent Olver for her hours of dedication counting up all those calories. Thank you to Carole Ann Rice for her enduring optimism. And, above all, thank you to the thousands of 'Jane Planners' out there who have lost weight and kept it off – you are my inspiration.

INTRODUCTION

TWENTY-TWO YEARS AGO, like you, I was trying to lose weight. It wasn't the first time I'd dieted. I must have been on dozens of diets over the course of my life, but this was to be the last. I lost more than 2 stone (12.7kg) and kept it off. Yes, 22 years later I am the same weight as I was immediately after that diet. I loved feeling slimmer, healthier and more in control. It changed the way I saw myself, and how others saw me, for the better. But, most importantly, for the first time I realised that the real secret to losing weight and keeping it off is simple – you just have to eat less and move more. Dieting doesn't have to be complicated or miserable, you *can* shift unwanted pounds and eat a range of gorgeous foods, as long as you watch your calories. Sounds obvious? It is.

As you and I both know, however, what's complicated is putting that philosophy into practice. That's why I came up with the Jane Plan Diet, which delivers calorie-counted, portion-controlled meals direct to the door so that all you have to do is eat them. You don't have to do anything else.

I wanted to combine my love of good food and healthy eating with my hard-earned knowledge of what it takes to lose weight and also how to keep it off – and, most importantly, what it's like to go on that journey. I knew from my own experience that if the meals were there, ready prepared, the rest would be a doddle. And that's exactly what Jane Plan is – borne out by the many thousands of people who have already succeeded in losing weight the Jane Plan way.

Why this book? I quickly realised that not everyone looking to lose weight wants food delivered to their door. You may like sourcing fresh, healthy ingredients for yourself as well as cooking. Many Jane Planners also told me that they were often lost for ideas about what to cook *after* they had reached their weight-loss goal and their Jane Plan delivery stopped coming. They wanted recipes and inspiration to keep them going on their new Jane Plan way of life.

I decided it was time for a DIY Jane Plan Diet and the result is this book. In the pages that follow you will learn the principles that have made Jane Plan so successful and how to put them into practice. No gimmicks. No false promises. Just simple-to-follow, down-to-earth, easy-to-stick-to advice, plus some yummy calorie-counted, portion-controlled recipes especially devised in the Jane Plan kitchen to ensure that this time you lose weight and keep it off – for ever.

Of course, it does require a bit more planning and organisation than having meals delivered direct to your door, but you'll find plenty of tips to help you on your way and to make everything as easy as possible. And because you can't cook all the time, you'll also find lots of ideas for quick and easy ways to follow Jane Plan with ready-prepared foods from your local supermarket or favourite lunch-time pit stop.

Before you turn the page, however, it's time for a bit of straight talking. To lose weight and keep it off you will have to change your eating habits, practise portion caution and start to balance your diet as well as your lifestyle. But it will be worth it. Losing weight will improve how you look and how you feel, as well as your overall health.

You probably know all these things already, but this book will help you to put that knowledge into practice. It will transform your life – your confidence will increase as well as your energy levels as the pounds drop off. Of course, there will be difficult moments but, with the strategies I'm going to give you, it will become easier – I promise.

Just imagine: you could be 1 stone (6.3kg) lighter in no time at all. Even better, you will keep that stone (or more) off for the rest of your life. Losing weight the Jane Plan way means losing weight *for ever*. So what are you waiting for? Let's get going. I will be with you on every page with hints and tips to keep you on the straight and narrow, encouraging you on your weight-loss journey.

JANE PLAN - HOW IT BEGAN

When a friend asked me why, despite always being on a 'diet', she never seemed to lose weight and how I managed to stay so slim, I asked her what and how much she was eating. Her answer was quite vague, so I decided to give her everything she needed to eat in one week – no more, no less – and to see what happened.

I popped into Waitrose, did a week's shop for her, wrote her a menu, including precise measurements of things such as how much cereal she should have for breakfast, while making sure that as much as possible was already

→

portion controlled. I arrived on her doorstep and told her to eat what I had given her – no more, no less – and to write everything down.

Lo and behold, the following week she had dropped 4 pounds (1.8kg), so we did it again, and again – and one month later she was 12 pounds (5.4kg) lighter. Her success made me realise that when it came to losing weight there was a real need for a helping hand. And that's how Jane Plan was born.

It sounds simple, but giving people exactly what they need to eat takes the hard work out of dieting. There's no guesswork, no shopping, no planning, no counting of points or meetings to attend. That's why Jane Plan is so easy.

Now, three years later and with thousands more successful weight-loss stories under my belt, I have decided it is time to bring the principles of Jane Plan to a wider audience.

HOW TO USE THIS BOOK

Whether you are looking for a healthy-eating plan or just want to lose weight, the Jane Plan Diet is designed to help you reach your goal and stick with it for life.

Part One: Get Started

Before you start out on your weight-loss journey, learn why being in the right frame of mind and setting goals is so important, as well as understanding how your body loses weight, how crucial it is to count calories and how to work out your ideal weight-loss goal.

Part Two: The Skinny Rules

Now you know the principles of weight loss, it is time to put your knowledge into practice with the eight Skinny Rules. The foundation of the Jane Plan Diet, these rules will teach you how to eat and live your life the slimmer way.

Part Three: Inside the Jane Plan Kitchen

Here you will find described the foods you will be eating, the menu planners, store-cupboard essentials and calorie charts, plus quick-and-easy recipes devised especially for you in the Jane Plan kitchen. There are also lots of tips on what to serve alongside the recipes.

Part Four: No Going Back

Life post-diet can be daunting, so this part shows you just how easy it is to keep weight off for good, if you stick to the basic Jane Plan principles.

LISTEN TO JANE'S TOP TIPS

To accompany this book you will find a free audio download of Jane's top tips for staying on track at www.janeplan.com/toptipsdownload

Part One

GET STARTED

Any kind of change you make in your life is as much about having the right mindset as it is about the actions you take. Before you start on your weight-loss journey, it's vital to get your head in the right place. Preparation and organisation are key not just in terms of making sure you have the right foods on hand to make changing your diet easy but in all kinds of other ways as well. How often have you started a diet full of good intentions only to find after a day or two that you have not been able to stick to it and are back to square one? Maybe you had not given enough thought to exactly why you wanted to lose weight, or perhaps other commitments got in the way? Or it's possible you didn't really understand that you do have to make some changes and conscious decisions to keep yourself on track.

→

This time is going to be different, because I have years of experience helping people lose weight successfully and I am going to give you all the help you need to set goals and focus on the lifestyle changes that will help you stick to your diet – and sustain your weight loss.

Before you try to change something, it's good to know why you're making a change, what needs to change and how to make it happen. Thinking long and hard about why you want to lose weight, and focusing on the benefits, will help motivate you. Keeping a food diary in which you record what you eat and drink can help you identify the specific areas of your diet that need addressing. Meanwhile, learning exactly how your body loses weight and why counting calories has such a crucial role to play will help to get the ball rolling. If you do things the Jane Plan way, losing weight need not be an uphill battle – and, best of all, this time you will keep off the pounds for good.

Chapter One

■

ENTER THE ZONE

YOU PROBABLY CAN'T WAIT to get started on the Jane Plan way of eating (when I ask people when they'd like to start their diet, many of them say 'immediately'). But although it's great to get going as soon as possible, it's important first to give some serious thought as to why you want to lose weight. Only you can decide what will motivate you to stick to a weight-loss plan, so think long and hard.

When the going gets tough (imagine being offered a comforting chocolate brownie, after a long day – hard to resist, right?), knowing exactly why you want to lose weight could make the difference between success and failure. You wouldn't start any new important project, either at work or at home, without knowing why you were doing it – so I urge you to give your reasons why serious thought.

Consider all the benefits of being slimmer. If it's just about looking better, that's fine, but bear in mind that according to psychologists if appearance is your only motivation you are less likely to succeed in the long run, so try to identify other reasons, such as health and emotional well-being. Everyone will have their own reason for wanting to lose weight: it might be seeing an unflattering photo of yourself, or your clothes no longer fitting, or you think you would feel more confident being slimmer, or perhaps your doctor has pointed out that you need to lose some weight.

You may have several reasons – that's fine. It's OK if it's for an upcoming event, such as a wedding, summer party or a beach holiday, but these could turn out to be quick fixes unless you look further ahead. Let's face it, you don't want to have to go on a diet every time something appears in your diary.

Try to go for a mixture of short-, medium- and long-term goals. Short-term goals will keep you focused from day to day, while medium-term goals will help give you a sense of achievement. This can keep you going when the end seems a long way off.

ALERT YOURSELF

Make a list of the things that are going to keep you focused – perhaps a photo of yourself, an encouraging phrase or sentence, or a picture of yourself when you were slimmer – and keep it around the house or your workplace where you can see it throughout the day, especially in moments of weakness and temptation. Set up alerts on your smart phone or reminders on your computer. Anything that reminds you of your weight-loss goals should do the trick.

GET *SMART*

Weight-loss attempts often fail because goals are unrealistic or too difficult to stick to. When planning goals, the secret is to make them SMART. This helps to ensure they are sustainable in the long term and stay that way. Many of you will have read about or used SMART goals before, but before you roll your eyes and think, Been there and done that, remember they are used so often for good reason: they work!

SMART goals are:

Specific Think about exactly what you want to achieve. Specify how much weight you want to lose and break it down into bite-sized manageable chunks; for example, start with an initial goal of losing 1 stone (6.3kg), then identify further goals, say 1½ stone (9.5kg), 2 stone (12.7kg), 2½ stone (15.8kg), 3 stone (19kg), and so on, until you have reached your ultimate goal. You can use this technique for dress size, waist measurement and even BMI (see page 39) – whichever works best for you.

To be Specific you also need to identify an end date. Each little goal needs to have a deadline, as well as the ultimate goal.

Measurable You will only know if you are achieving your goals if you can measure them, so, for example, rather than saying you are going to eat less to lose weight, decide how many calories you are going to eat a day (I will show you how to work this out on pages 46–50), exactly what you are going to eat, and when you are going to eat. Then, write it down. Keeping an accurate food diary is the best way to do this, as I explain on pages 31–7.

The same principle can be applied to activities. Rather than saying that you are going to exercise more, decide how long you are going to walk for, where and on how many days; for example, you could decide to walk for 20 minutes every day at lunchtime. Make a note on your calendar, mobile or other device just as you would for any other appointment so that you can tick it off.

Achievable To be successful, goals must take into account your current situation; for example, think about your forthcoming schedule – do you have a holiday planned? Do you have to eat out for work several times over the next few weeks? Have you decided to diet from Monday through to Friday only and take the weekends off? If any of these apply, you need to understand that although your goal is still achievable, your weight loss will be slower.

Also, consider your fitness level, any health niggles and how much time you have available. Tailoring your goals to suit your lifestyle helps you set goals that are sustainable and therefore achievable.

Realistic Being realistic about what you can and can't achieve is also important; for example, it is probably not realistic to aim for a size 8 if you have never been anywhere near that dress size since you were a teenager. It is much better to set a more realistic goal of getting to a size 14 or 12. You can always revise it downwards once you have reached that size.

Time specific It's no good saying, 'I will start eating the Jane Plan way in a week or two.' You need to choose a definite start date for your weight-loss journey, note it somewhere and stick to it. Remember that the sooner you start, the sooner you will reach your goal. In the next chapter I explain how setting a start date will help you to prepare mentally for success with your diet.

Review your progress each week. Did you successfully meet your goals? Think about what worked and what didn't, and why. Don't beat yourself up if you slip up occasionally, simply make a mental note of what happened and why, then plan how to avoid it the following week.

BEWARE: YOUR GOALS CAN CHANGE

You may need to change or re-think a goal after a few weeks; for example, perhaps you started small and are ready for a bigger challenge, or perhaps something has changed in your life, such as your job or relationship, and you need to adjust your goals accordingly.

I often talk with people who change their goals as they lose weight. Interestingly, some start off wanting to lose 3 stone (19kg), but when they reach the 2 stone (12.7kg) mark they are happy to stick with it. On the other hand, others reach their goal weight and then decide they'd like to lose more.

WHAT TYPE OF EATER ARE YOU?

Identifying what type of eater you are can help pinpoint your weak points, making it easier to see areas that need addressing. This is all about putting you in the driving seat. Knowing what makes you overeat enables you to put measures in place to combat it. The act of eating is often about more than just hunger – and when we *overeat* it can be because we are bored, depressed, we don't want to say no, or a host of other reasons. Once you know what type of eater you are, you can stop eating too much, too often and the wrong things.

Do you fit any of the patterns in the chart overleaf?

WHAT TYPE OF EATER ARE YOU?

Type	Signs	Fight-back tactics
Bored eater/ unconscious eater	You eat without paying attention to your food. You eat when bored at your desk, in the car or in front of the TV. You are never aware of, or remember, what or how much you are eating. You pay little attention to when you are eating and aren't aware of when you are full. You eat on the run and often while standing up	Ban food from the car and your desk, and only eat in the kitchen or dining room. No more TV dinners. Follow the Jane Plan rule: never eat standing up or on the run; sit down every time you eat. Write down everything you eat and drink – keep a food diary. Sign up to My Fitness Pal
Comfort eater	You turn to food to make yourself feel happier and better about yourself, but it often has the reverse effect, leaving you feeling guilty and depressed. After a bad day at work or a row with a loved one you turn to food for comfort. You tend to binge. You turn to food when you feel lonely or sad and see food as your friend. You crave chocolate when depressed	Avoid the kitchen. Have a long, relaxing bath (a great de-stressor). Go for a walk (exercise releases endorphins that make you feel good). Phone a friend. Go shopping online and buy that dress – it could make you feel better about yourself. Light a scented candle. Relax on the sofa with a trashy magazine. Lose yourself in a great book. Distract yourself by painting your nails or doing a home pedicure

Type	Signs	Fight-back tactics
People pleaser	You're too embarrassed to turn food down or to say no, or you don't want to draw attention to the fact that you are trying to lose weight. You can't say no to food for fear of offending family or friends. You feel socially obliged to eat and drink what everyone else is eating and drinking, especially at business lunches	Don't be afraid to ring up your host ahead of a family party to say you are watching your portions. When eating out in a restaurant, go for the lower-calorie options and don't feel obliged to indulge in every course, just because your friends are. At business lunches leave before the pudding – say you have another meeting to attend
Abundant eater	You are always in the kitchen creating something delicious. You just love food. Your portions are out of control	Ban baking. Biscuits and cakes are the downfall of many a good cook; once baked, who can resist? Focus on healthy ingredients and be creative with vegetables and salads. Avoid cooking too many sauces. Ditch the desserts – opt for fruit salads, sorbets or granita

➜

Type	Signs	Fight-back tactics
Weekend indulger/ treater	You are a model dieter Monday to Friday, even if you are super-stressed and super-busy! But at weekends you reward yourself for being so good and over-indulge. Friday-night takeaways, Saturday-morning fry-ups and Sunday lunches feature high on the weekend menu	A couple of weekend treats won't undo the week's hard work, but overdoing it every weekend will. Throw away takeaway menus – out of sight out of mind. Enjoy long, lazy brunches, and indulge in exotic fruit, scrambled eggs and smoked salmon. There's no place for a fry-up on Jane Plan. Don't take the whole weekend off – if you really feel the need to take time out from Jane Plan, have one splurge night a week instead
Fast-food junky/ ready-meal muncher	Your life is hectic and stressful, so you have no time to shop, cook and eat healthily. You live on ready meals and pre-prepared food. You grab a sandwich for lunch and snack on crisps and chocolate	Plan your week and shop ahead. Cook in bulk at the weekend and pop individual portions in the freezer for weekdays. Try online shopping. Become an avid label reader – ready meals are often high in fat and calories

Type	Signs	Fight-back tactics
Celebratory eater	At a party or event you tend to overeat and drink at the buffet or table – it's too hard to resist	Try to focus on the social aspect of the event rather than the canapés. Ignore the wine and champagne. Go for a glass of water or a spritzer
Naughty nibbler	You graze throughout the day. You're constantly checking out the contents of the fridge. You nibble off the children's plates. You eat standing up or walking along the street	Ban the biscuit tin. Only keep fresh, healthy food in the fridge. Hide the crisps and other nibble-type foods – even better, don't have them in the house. Don't keep sweets or biscuits in your desk drawer
Plate piler	You eat huge portions. You rarely eat between meals, but you pile your plate high at table. You overeat in the evening and stand at the fridge munching	Eat regularly through the day: breakfast, lunch and dinner. Stick to two snacks a day between meals. Don't sit down for dinner starving – eat crudités before dinner. Drink a large glass of water before eating

There is even more information to help you understand your eating patterns and how you can change them in the Skinny Rules in Part Two.

Chapter Two

■

SET A DATE AND GET STARTED

MAKING UP YOUR MIND to go on a diet can be difficult, but starting and sticking to it can be even harder. Let's face it, there is never a good moment. What's more, it is easy to make excuses that get in the way of taking that first step. Every day hundreds of people tell me the reasons they never got round to starting a diet, and the reasons are usually similar:

'I'm too busy right now; I'll wait until things calm down.'

'I just love food and can't bear the thought of life without being able to eat what I want.'

'I can't see the point – the weight will just pile back on as soon as I finish.'

'Eating healthily costs too much.'

'I'll start when the children are back at school/after my holiday/ when the house renovations have finished.'

These are just some of the hundreds of excuses people use. Typical excuses, perhaps, but the bottom line is that you *can* make time, you *can* have the occasional naughty food – you won't put the weight back on if you start to eat the Jane Plan way, and it *doesn't* have to cost the earth.

Starting a diet is really not that bad. In fact, it can actually be enjoyable. People frequently tell me how relieved they are once they have started, how they enjoy the feeling of being in control and how satisfying it is to see results. The secret is to focus on your goals and approach your diet in an unemotional way; for example, the same way you would on a work project: no matter how painful it is, or how many long hours you are going to have to spend in the office while your friends are out having fun, you just have to get on with it. Delaying it will only make it harder in the long run, but doing it well could lead to a promotion or a pay rise. And remember: the job that never gets started never gets finished.

If you're a stay-at-home mum, approach your diet in the same way you would 'homework time'. I remember trying to get my tired eight-year-old started on his homework, when he'd rather be watching TV. I'd try to explain that it had to be done, and that the sooner he started the better, and who knows, he might actually enjoy it. Of course, once he'd actually started, it didn't seem quite so bad. It might not have been his first choice of how to spend his evening, but he knew he had to do it and, after a bit of encouragement, he'd finally get going. He also knew that the longer he left it, the worse it would become, and the more tired he would be. Sound familiar?

Well, imagine your diet is either your homework or your work project; it's not what you want to do, you know it might involve some sacrifices, but it's better to start sooner rather than later, and you're going to reap the benefits in the long term. A new, slimmer you!

Just as you tell the children it's important that they do their homework to help them get on in the world, it's important to tell yourself the same. They may prefer to watch *Doctor Who* than do homework, and you may prefer a chocolate muffin to a healthy salad, but at some point you just have to say NO and get on with it.

There's never a 'right' time. You've just got to take the plunge, make a date and stick with it. Putting a start date on your calendar or setting up an alert on your smartphone can help, as psychologically they signify change.

Before getting started, it's wise to look in your kitchen cupboards and see what foods are going to scupper your diet efforts.

DETOX YOUR KITCHEN

When you are trying to lose weight, or even just to eat healthily, your kitchen, with its cupboards and fridge brimming with tempting treats, can become your worst enemy. The secret is to give it a quick detox before you take that first important step. Tidying and decluttering can also help to put you in the right mindset for your weight-loss journey. You may well be amazed at how much rubbish you have squirrelled away, and you may even be relieved to see the back of it.

Jane Wisdom

Don't start your diet until you have thrown away all tempting treats – the foods that could make you stray – and that includes those takeaway menus. Remember: 'Better in the bin than in the belly!'

Hide away tempting treats You eat with your eyes rather than your stomach, so you are much more likely to reach for naughty foods if they are visible. Hide them at the back of your cupboards or in sealed tins or boxes: out of sight, out of mind. Better still, get rid of them – the temptation of opening a pack or jar may be too hard to resist. Give your fridge and freezer a good going over and don't forget those bottles of wine. Take them out of the fridge and put them at the back of a cupboard or, if you are lucky enough to have one, in the cellar.

Keep healthy foods visible Did you know that research shows you are three times more likely to eat the first thing you see in the kitchen than the fifth? Move healthy options to the front of the fridge or cupboard so that they stare you in the face as you open the door. Keep fruit bowls filled with plenty of fresh fruit and ready-chopped crudités in the fridge. That way there's always something handy for you to snack on.

Re-organise your dishes and plates Research shows that you are likely to eat 40 per cent more from a large plate of a given amount of food than from a smaller plate or bowl containing the same amount. You are also more likely to serve yourself a larger portion on a larger plate, so keep small plates and bowls at the front of the cupboard for quick, easy access. Wrap up large plates in tissue paper and store them at the back or on top of the cupboard well out of reach.

Divide glasses into two sections It is easier to drink faster and more from short, fat glasses, so keep these for daytime hydration, to quench your thirst. For the evening go for tall, thin glasses. The reason? Studies show you are more likely to sip more slowly and drink less from them.

Get positive It can be tempting to open the fridge door and give in to temptation, so why not transform your fridge door into a positive reminder of your weight-loss goals? Stick up some inspirational quotes or a photo of yourself that you really love as well as a list of five reasons why you aren't going to give in.

SHOP WITH CARE

Eating the Jane Plan way starts with the food you buy – and making the right choice at the supermarket can make all the difference between success and failure.

Make a list Healthy decisions start at home, so always make a list before you brave the supermarket aisles, and don't deviate from it. Planning your meals for the week ahead, and the ingredients you will need, reduces the risk of you straying towards those tempting but less healthy foods. It will also save time and money.

Beware of abundance shopping Don't be influenced by supermarket selling strategies. It's your decision what you buy – not theirs. BOGOFs (buy one get one free) or buy three for the price of two might seem appealing, but think about it: do you really need three punnets of strawberries or eight apples instead of four? The more you have, the greater the chance of them ending up in your stomach or the bin. Eating the Jane Plan way means buying higher quality food in smaller amounts.

Jane Wisdom
Remember: what you buy dictates what you eat.

Jane Wisdom

Over-buying increases the risk of overeating – you can always pop down to your local shop if you run out of anything.

DID YOU KNOW?

The average person throws away £480 worth of food a year. It is not only wasteful but it is also bad for the environment.

Avoid shopping with the children Don't underestimate the influence of 'pester' power. You could end up with more in your shopping trolley than you either bargained or budgeted for. If you do end up with the children pulling at your purse strings, the rule is: mentally distinguish between what you need, what you want and what you fancy.

Get aisle wise Give centre supermarket aisles a miss. The reason? That's where those tempting naughty foods like to lurk. Instead, linger longer in the outer aisles, which usually house the fresh fruit and veg sections. Sticking to supermarket outskirts will also help you avoid impulse snack buys.

Don't shop when hungry Everything will look twice as appealing, making it far harder to resist those naughty nibbles. If you do find yourself in the supermarket with an empty stomach, buying and drinking a bottle of water or chomping on a piece of fresh fruit can help to quell those hunger pangs.

Be a label reader Compare similar foods and check out serving sizes, calories, fat, cholesterol and salt content. Go for the one that's lower in fat, but make sure it's also lower in calories – low-fat and fat-free foods can be calorie high.

Which eating habits do you need to change?

Over the years, bad eating habits can creep up without you realising. Try this quiz to help identify yours and read on to discover what you can do to break the pattern.

	Yes	No
1. Do you always eat everything on your plate?	☐	☐
2. Do you eat the same amount as your husband or teenage son?	☐	☐
3. If thirsty, do you reach for some juice rather than a bottle of water?	☐	☐
4. Do you eat on the run or graze throughout the day?	☐	☐
5. Are you always the first to finish your food?	☐	☐
6. Is a sandwich your usual weekday lunch?	☐	☐
7. Is a mid-morning cappuccino and pastry part of your daily routine?	☐	☐
8. Is a glass of wine an occasional treat or more of an every evening event?	☐	☐

Changing habits can be one of the hardest challenges when it comes to losing weight, but if you answered yes to any of these questions, it's time to have a re-think for the sake of your waist-line. But before you sink into despondency, making changes the Jane Plan way won't disrupt your lifestyle that much and, best of all, you will be able to sustain them in the long term.

MAKE CHANGES NOW

1. If you always chomp though everything on your plate, slow down and focus carefully on each mouthful. Most of us have grown up with the belief that we should finish all the food we are given, but eating the Jane Plan way means becoming conscious about the amount you eat, and being more in control. It's good practice to leave a little food on your plate. That way *you* are in control, *you* are choosing exactly how much you eat, not the person who served the meal.

2. Women simply can't afford to eat the same as the men in the family. The reason? Men are taller and more muscular, and have a higher metabolic rate, meaning they can burn off calories faster. Sadly, when it comes to weight loss, not all things are equal.

3. Juice may have more allure than water, but it is generally loaded with calories and sugar – even the smallest bottle can contain as many as 80 calories. The secret is to carry a water bottle with you at all times.

Jane Wisdom
Thirsty people tend to eat more.

4. Do you eat on the run – and often with your fingers? If so, it's easy to forget what you have eaten as well as forgetting to count the calories. Make a rule that you will always sit down to eat and use a knife, fork and spoon.

5. Always being the first at the table to finish your food is bad for your digestion and makes you more likely to succumb to second helpings. The advice in point 1 on page 25 applies here too. Research suggests that it takes about 20 minutes for your brain to register that you are full, so taking your time allows your brain to catch up with the signals coming from your digestive system.

6. Often sandwiches are high in calories and typical fillings are high in fat and salt. It's time to stop buying workday lunches on autopilot and broaden your repertoire. Sushi, readymade salads or soup (without the bread), for example, are much healthier options and widely available at most popular sandwich shops as well as supermarkets.

7. An apple gives you more va-va-voom than a coffee. Avoid fluctuating sugar levels and ditch the cappuccino and pastry mid-morning in favour of a piece of fruit. Keep it in your desk drawer, in your handbag – wherever is most convenient for you. If you feel you need a hot drink, green tea will give you that much-needed caffeine hit.

8. The dangers of 'wine o'clock' are well documented. If you find yourself on autopilot to the fridge or the bar after a long, hard day, think again. Alcohol damages not only your diet but also your health, and can make stress levels even higher. Find something else to calm you down and help you relax.

SWAP IT

Breakfast

▶ Swap whole milk for semi-skimmed, 1 per cent fat or even skimmed milk.

▶ Swap a sugar-coated breakfast cereal for wholegrain muesli, porridge or granola with no added sugar. (Choose carefully, even the healthiest-looking mueslis and granolas can be laden with calories – avoid those with too much dried fruit; also remember that a ramekin portion size – 57 × 25mm – is enough.)

▶ Swap full-fat or sweetened yoghurt for lower-fat or fat-free Greek yoghurt, or natural low-fat yoghurt.

▶ Swap bacon for eggs, and sausages for grilled tomatoes and mushrooms.

▶ Swap boiled egg and soldiers for boiled egg and spinach or asparagus, or broccoli spears.

▶ Swap a smoothie for a piece of fruit and a glass of water.

Lunch

▶ Swap bread for oatcakes.

▶ Swap sandwiches for sushi or soup.

▶ Swap pasta salads or other salads with mayonnaise for fresh green or mixed salads.

▶ Swap a plate of pasta for a bowl of soup (without the bread).

→

▶ Swap cheese, ham or tuna mayonnaise for smoked salmon, hummus, cottage cheese or tzatziki.

Dinner

▶ Swap creamy or cheesy sauces for tomato- or vegetable-based sauces.

▶ Swap salad dressing for a squeeze of lemon or lime juice – adding a sprinkling seeds to salads can also enhance the flavour.

▶ Swap fatty meats for leaner cuts and remove the skin – even better, eat more fish.

▶ Swap pasta for courgette spaghetti (page 237) and rice for cauliflower rice (page 239). If that's too much faff, just double up on your vegetable portion.

▶ Swap the frying pan for the grill or, even better, steam cook where possible.

▶ Swap butter for olive oil.

▶ Swap salt for seasoning and use fresh herbs or even chilli.

▶ Swap desserts for fresh fruit.

Drinks

▶ Swap a coffee made with whole milk to a 'skinny' coffee made with semi-skimmed or skimmed milk, or even better, a herbal tea.

→

▶ Swap standard squash for a squash with no added sugars.

▶ Swap juices for water.

Snacks

▶ Swap a blueberry muffin for an oatcake with a teaspoon of honey.

▶ Swap biscuits for a very small handful of nuts (6–9 is about the right amount, depending on the nut – check out our Mini Mouthfuls list, page 147, for more info on nuts).

▶ Swap crisps for crudités.

▶ Swap sweets and chocolate for fruit.

Chapter Three

■

WRITE IT DOWN

'I SWEAR I DON'T EAT A LOT, so why do I weigh so much?', 'Diets never work for me – I never seem to lose weight, although I stick to the plan.' These are just a couple of cries I regularly hear from people as they think about starting to eat the Jane Plan way. I suspect the reason for their groans is that they are simply not aware of exactly what they are eating or, just as importantly, how much they are eating, whether it's the amount they are piling on their plates or the nibbles they are sneaking in between meals. In most cases they simply don't know, and if they do they dare not admit it – even to themselves.

Jane Wisdom
If you eat on the run, you'll forget you've eaten at all.

Let's face it, it is easy to go from day to day kidding yourself that certain things don't really count – either because no one can see you eating them or because you think they are so small that they won't make any difference to your weight anyway. Of course, it can be hard to keep track of every morsel, but it is not impossible.

DIARY IT – WHAT, WHEN AND WITH WHOM?

The best way to keep track of what you are eating is to keep a food diary in which you note down every single thing you eat and drink, when you consume it and with whom.

It's an approach that is amply backed by science. Research shows that keeping a food diary can double the amount of weight you lose on a diet. In fact, research published in the *American Journal of Preventive Medicine* showed that people keeping a food diary six days a week lost about twice as much weight as those who kept a diary for one day a week or less. Make a resolution to keep a diary – and stick to it.

Jane Wisdom

Keeping a food diary will not only help you lose weight but it will also help you to keep it off.

Here's how to get started:

▶ Buy or make yourself a food diary. One that fits into the back pocket of your jeans is often the best, as it is always close to hand. But if you're into technology, you can use your mobile, and there are even apps you can use to keep track of your daily food intake.

▶ Keep your diary with you all the time and write down everything you eat as you eat it. You are more likely to be honest if you write it in as you go rather than filling it in retrospectively. It's too easy to forget that bar of chocolate or piece of cake that you sneaked in – the ones that can make all the difference between success and failure.

▶ Be very specific; for example, what size was your cappuccino? Did you have two or three oatcakes? And how many glasses of wine did you down? Was it one, two or even three? Did you have chicken with the skin on or off? Were your potatoes roasted or boiled? Did you add gravy? Remember, every single detail counts.

▶ Always note the time, the place and how you were feeling when you were eating.

▶ Don't make any exceptions. Water, chewing gum, and even the odd Polo mint, all count.

▶ If you miss recording a meal or two, don't beat yourself up. Every entry you make is taking you one step closer to a better understanding of your food choices and habits.

A food diary can help you lose weight because:

▶ The very action of writing something down is often enough to stop you putting food in your mouth.

▶ It instantly makes you more aware of what, how much and why you are eating, which can help to reduce mindless munching.

► It will identify areas that need addressing, which will help you on your weight-loss journey.

► It will help you understand your relationship with food, especially if you note down what and how you were feeling before, during and after eating.

► Looking back at weeks when you have felt satisfied and lost weight can keep you motivated and on track, especially if you feel challenged one week.

► You will eat less as you become more conscious of your habits.

► It can help you recognise triggers to avoid, such as starving yourself all day then stuffing yourself at night.

You diary will also record your weight-loss progress and the exercise you have taken.

WEIGHING YOURSELF — IT'S ESSENTIAL TO BE CONSISTENT

Keeping track of your weight also requires 100 per cent honesty. Perhaps you are tempted to cheat on the scales, perhaps by moving them to a different place in the hope of getting a different reading, or maybe you are too scared of what your true weight might be to get on them in the first place. But cheating or avoiding the truth will only keep you where you are, and that's exactly where you don't want to be.

So come on, pluck up your courage and hop on those scales. Once you know the truth, you have something to work with, and keeping a note of your weight from week to week is a great way of staying motivated and on track.

Here's how to be accurate:

▶ Weigh yourself on the same scales in the same place once a week rather than every day. Weight varies from day to day (which may be due to water retention or a higher carb meal the night before, which can also cause you to retain water) and an unfavourable reading can be demotivating. What happens to demotivated dieters? They dive head first into the biscuit tin.

▶ If you get a weigh-in result you aren't happy with, don't move the scales around the room hoping for a different result! You'll probably get one, but consistency is the key to success here.

▶ Make sure the battery is up to scratch – old batteries give inconsistent results.

▶ Decide exactly what time you are going to weigh yourself and stick to it every week.

▶ You'll weigh more in the evening than in the morning.

▶ It's best to weigh yourself as soon as you get up, in the morning, with no clothes on. Post-poo is best. If that's not going to work for you – be consistent. Decide to do it pre- or post-poo and stick to your decision.

▶ If you can't weigh in naked, make sure you are wearing the same clothes each week. If you wear boots, jeans and a belt one week, you'll get a very different result the next week if you are wearing a chiffon dress.

▶ Note down your weekly weight in your food diary. It can be incredibly motivating to chart your weight loss from week to week.

▶ Constipation could also skew your weigh-in.

▶ For women, weighing in just before (or in the early stages of) your period may not give you a good result. Don't worry – it's completely normal to retain water during that time of the month. The good news is that next week you'll see a positive result again.

Jane Wisdom
Digital bathroom scales will give you a more accurate reading than the old-fashioned spring-balance type.

HOW TO SET OUT YOUR FOOD DIARY

Overleaf there is an example of what an ideal food diary looks like. Include lots of detail.

At the end of the food diary you will find an example of how to record your activities. Keeping a record of how active you are every day and for how long can help you to establish a regular exercise routine as well as keeping your motivation high. For ideas on how to move more see Skinny Rule 8 on page 111. And don't forget to weigh yourself at the same time every week, naked or wearing the same clothes.

HOW TO SET OUT A FOOD DIARY

Date:	What did you eat?	What did you drink?	How did you feel?	Who were you with?
Breakfast	Ramekin (57 x 25mm) of muesli, 100ml of skimmed milk. Handful of strawberries	Cup of Earl Grey tea. Splash of skimmed milk	Great!	The children
Snack	An apple	Cup of coffee. Splash of skimmed milk	A bit sleepy until I had my coffee	By myself
Lunch	½ tub of cottage cheese. Handful of rocket, 2 tomatoes, 8 slices of cucumber, 1 peach	2 glasses of water	Fine – didn't need the peach, but I'm used to having something sweet after a meal	Friends at work
Snack	3 dried apricots, Small piece of fish finger left over from the children's tea	Cup of Earl Grey. Splash of skimmed milk	Low on energy, wanted to nibble at the kids' tea	By myself

			My partner
Dinner	3 tbsp chilli con carne – no rice but a handful of broccoli, handful of mangetouts	Small glass of wine, 3 glasses of fizzy mineral water	Wanted a lot more wine! Stressful day – very hungry before dinner
Portions of fruit and vegetables	5–6		
Any other snacks	3 Polos in the car when picking the kids up from school		Wanted to nibble before dinner – will prepare crudités for tomorrow to nibble while preparing dinner
Any other drinks		1 litre of water, 2 diet cokes	

Exercise	How long?	How did you feel?
Walking	30 minutes	A bit tired, but invigorated

Date	Weight	Loss/change
1 January	11st 5lb	-2lb

Chapter Four

■

UNDERSTANDING WEIGHT LOSS

BEFORE YOU START the Jane Plan way of eating, you also
need to understand how your body loses weight. There
are so many different theories that it is not surprising
many of us are confused. I am going to cut through the myths
and show you that actually it's not that complicated. Don't
worry, I'm not going to blind you with scientific facts and
figures, but I am going to help you understand the importance
of counting calories.

How often have you said to yourself, 'Why haven't I lost
a pound when I've been really good? I don't understand it',
or 'I haven't eaten a thing all week, yet I have put on weight'?
Understanding how your body works means that you will
know why that has happened and you will never need to ask
those questions again. You'll know the answers and you'll find
losing weight so much easier.

What weight should you be aiming for?

Before explaining the importance of calorie counting on your weight-loss journey you need to find out what is a healthy weight for you. A healthy body mass index (BMI) is 20–24.9. If you have a BMI above the healthy range, you are at raised risk of the serious health problems linked to being overweight, such as heart disease, type-2 diabetes and certain cancers. But see below, because not all people with higher BMIs are unhealthy.

Use the simple table overleaf to find your ideal weight range. Once you have reached your ideal weight you will not only look and feel better, but will also be healthier.

For a healthy BMI of 20–24.9 the weight and height ranges shown in the table apply.

(You can also use the chart on the NHS Livewell pages – www.nhs.uk/livewell/healthy-living/pages/height-weight-chart.aspx. Alternatively, visit janeplan.com.)

What is a 'healthy' BMI?

BMI below 20: with a score this low you may be underweight.

BMI from 20–24.9: this is a healthy range.

BMI of 25 or more: your BMI is above the ideal range – you may be overweight.

BMI of 30 or more: a BMI of 30 is classified as obese.

Your BMI reading indicates how heavy you are for your height; however, because we are all built differently, and some of us may have more muscle mass than others, a BMI reading is not always the best indicator of body fat. Use the BMI as a guide, and if you are concerned, ask your doctor for help.

IDEAL WEIGHT RANGE FOR A HEALTHY BMI

Imperial measurement

Metric measurement

Height in feet and inches	Weight in stones/ pounds	Height in metres	Weight in kilos
4ft 8in	6st 5lb–8st 0lb	1.42m	40–51kg
4ft 9in	6st 8lb–8st 4lb	1.45m	42–53kg
4ft 10in	6st 12lb–8st 8lb	1.47m	44–54kg
4ft 11in	7st 1lb–8st 12lb	1.50m	45–56kg
5ft	7st 4lb–9st 2lb	1.52m	46–58kg
5ft 1in	7st 8lb–9st 6lb	1.55m	48–60kg
5 ft 2in	7st 11lb–9st 11lb	1.57m	49–62kg
5ft 3in	8st 1lb–10st 1lb	1.60m	51–64kg
5ft 4in	8st 5lb–10st 6lb	1.63m	53–66kg
5ft 5in	8st 8lb–10st 10lb	1.65m	54–68kg
5ft 6in	8st 12lb–11st 1lb	1.68m	56–70kg
5ft 7in	9st 2lb–11st 6lb	1.70m	58–73kg
5ft 8in	9st 6lb–11st 10lb	1.73m	60–74kg
5ft 9in	9st 9lb–12st 1lb	1.75m	61–77kg
5ft 10in	9st 13lb–12st 6lb	1.78m	63–79kg
5ft 11in	10st 3lb–12st 11lb	1.80m	65–81kg
6ft	10st 7lb–13st 2lb	1.83m	67–83kg
6ft 1in	10st 12lb–13st 7lb	1.85m	69–86kg
6ft 2in	11st 2lb–13st 13lb	1.88m	71–88kg
6ft 3in	11st 6lb–14st 4lb	1.91m	73–91kg
6ft 4in	11st 10lb–14st 9lb	1.93m	74–93kg
6ft 5in	12st 1lb–15st 1lb	1.96m	77–96kg
6ft 6in	12st 5lb–15st 7lb	1.98m	78–98kg
6ft 7in	12st 10lb–15st 12lb	2.00m	80–100kg

DO YOU MEASURE UP?

Measuring is another good way to find out whether you have healthy amounts of body fat.

A fit woman who is a size 12 might weigh more than an unfit woman who is the same clothing size, because the fit woman has more muscle mass. Measuring your waist circumference with a tape measure can give you a more accurate idea of how healthy you are than knowing your BMI, because it reflects the amount of fat around your vital organs. Use a flexible tape measure and measure your waist just above the highest points on your hipbone, while breathing normally – don't suck your stomach in.

According to the NHS, you have a higher risk of health problems if your waist size is:

More than 94cm (37in), if you're a man

More than 80cm (31.5in), if you're a woman

Your risk of health problems is even higher if your waist size is:

More than 102cm (40in), if you're a man

More than 88cm (34.5in), if you're a woman

Jane Wisdom
You will be regularly weighing in throughout your weight-loss journey, and it's a good idea to take your waist measurements at regular intervals too.

KNOW YOUR CALORIES

Now that you have established a healthy weight and waist size for you it's time to look at the best ways to drop any excess pounds. Ask any qualified nutritionist or dietitian for advice on how to do it and they'll give you the same answer: you need to create a calorie deficit. In other words, you need to take in fewer calories than you expend (or use) so that your body has to draw on its fat stores to provide energy. The result is you lose fat and the pounds fall away!

What's a calorie?

Now for a bit of science. We all use the word 'calorie' with abandon, but do you really know what calories are? I certainly didn't until I studied nutrition. To lose weight and keep it off in the long term you really need to get to grips with them. Basically, calories can be used to measure any type of energy, but they are usually associated with food. Scientifically, one calorie is the amount of energy needed to raise the temperature of 1g of water by 1°C. Nutritionally speaking, when you hear that something contains 100 calories, it's a way of describing how much energy your body could get from eating or drinking it.

Calories in vs calories out

With so many fad diets around and so much hype about losing weight, it can be easy to forget that weight is all about the balance between energy (calories) in – in other words, the food you eat – and energy (calories) out – in other words, how much you burn through activity, including going about your daily life. As I explained above, getting the balance right is what determines whether you will achieve your weight-loss goal.

Jane Wisdom
Following a calorie-controlled diet is the only guaranteed way to help you lose those unwanted pounds. The key to success is to know how many calories to eat.

Think of your energy balance a bit like your bank account. You make regular *deposits* when you eat or drink. You make *withdrawals* when your body burns up energy. The calories or energy you burn can be divided into two parts:

1. The energy your body needs to keep all your basic bodily functions going, known as your basal metabolic rate (BMR).

2. The energy you need over and above this to cover physical activity, known as your active metabolic rate (AMR).

Whenever you eat anything, your body takes what it needs to cover its outgoings and stores the rest as fat or glycogen, which is slowly converted into fat (think of it like putting aside savings for a rainy day). To keep your energy account in balance, just like your bank account, you need to take in enough each day to cover your basic outgoings. If you want to lose weight, however, you need to take in a little less so that your body is forced to tap into its savings of stored energy (that is, what it has laid down as fat).

Just as with your bank account, you don't have much control over how much you spend on your basic mortgage and bills; when it comes to your body, about 70 per cent of the energy you withdraw is out of your control; it's used to keep your internal organs – such as your heart and lungs – working. However, you do have some control over how much of the remaining amount you use, which can be increased by regular exercise.

Jane Wisdom

Eating the Jane Plan way gives you the opportunity to try out new things as you cut out the old.

It sounds simple, and it is, but before you decide how many calories you are going to allow yourself in order to achieve your weight-loss goal you need to know how many calories you are currently consuming in a day. In order to do this you need to work out your BMR. This will tell you how many calories you need each day to maintain your current weight when you are at rest (that is, assuming you stayed in bed all day).

First, let's look at the factors that affect your BMR and, in turn, your body's ability to lose weight.

Your weight and the effects of age, height, activity and gender

Age

Have you ever wondered why, as you get older, you seem to find it harder to lose weight? It's because your body becomes less efficient at burning calories. The reason? Muscles become weaker and smaller (the official term is atrophy), and as muscle is what experts call highly metabolically active – that is, it is super-efficient at burning calories – unless you take steps to maintain, or even build, muscle you need fewer daily calories.

For women, the bad news is that you experience this to a greater extent than men! As a result, around the time of the menopause, or even before, if you continue to eat the same way you did in your twenties and thirties, you will start to put on weight. To reverse it, you need to eat less, and/or embark on some serious resistance training.

Jane Wisdom
It can be mystifying when you put on weight after you turn 40, or post-menopause, even though you have not changed your diet, but the simple reason is that your body becomes less efficient at burning calories as you age.

Height

It's not just age that affects BMR; your overall size, including your height, also has a part to play. Taller and heavier people who have a larger percentage of muscle mass have a higher metabolic rate. In the same way as a double-decker bus waiting on the side of the road with its engine running will use more fuel than a small Mini, so a taller, heavier person is likely to lose weight faster than someone smaller and lighter. Such people are also in the lucky position of being able to eat more than a smaller, lighter person and still maintain their weight.

Activity

Needless to say, exercise also has a part to play. People who take a lot of exercise are likely to have a greater percentage of muscle tissue and, because muscle burns calories more efficiently than non-muscle tissue, those people are likely to have a higher BMR than non-muscly people.

Don't think that exercising gives you free licence to eat loads more, though. True, some types of exercise are more efficient calorie burners than others. (See Skinny Rule 8, page 111.) But cutting down the number of calories you consume is still the mainstay of weight loss.

Gender

Finally, have you ever wondered why men tend to lose weight faster than women? Unfair as it seems, the answer is that they tend to be taller, heavier and have a higher muscle mass, which means they have a higher BMR and so (generally) burn more calories than women.

Jane Wisdom

As you get older, it is harder to eat what you want and stay thin – that's because BMR decreases with age.

HOW TO WORK OUT YOUR BMR

Working out your BMR used to be tricky and time-consuming, but luckily technology has made it a whole lot simpler. There's now a host of online tools, apps and other devices that can work it out for you. You'll find Jane Plan's own BMR calculator at www.janeplan.com. All you have to do is enter your gender, weight, height and age to get your BMR, and the site will do the rest. You then include your activity levels to find out how many calories you need each day to maintain your current weight. Many digital bathroom scales do the same thing, so look out for that facility when buying a new set. Alternatively, you can calculate your BMR the old-fashioned way as explained in the box opposite.

CALCULATE YOUR BMR

You can work out your basal metabolic rate (BMR) by using something called the Harris Benedict equation. It is not as complicated as it may at first seem, so here's the formula if you want to give it a go. Unless you're a maths wizard you'll need to use a calculator.

BMR calculation for women:

655 + (4.35 × [your weight in pounds]) + (4.7 × [your height in inches]) – (4.7 × [your age in years])

BMR calculation for men:

66 + (6.23 × [your weight in pounds]) + (12.7 × [your height in inches]) – (6.76 × [your age in years])

Work out your daily calorie needs

To work out your total daily calorie requirement to maintain your current weight you now need to multiply your BMR with an appropriate activity multiplier. That's because your BMR only tells you how many calories you need to maintain your *current weight at rest* and, of course, you are unlikely to be lying in bed all day. Even if you aren't an avid gym bunny you will still be doing some sort of activity, even if it's just sitting at a desk.

Select the activity level that best describes you from the chart overleaf, and multiply your BMR by the activity multiplier. If you can't quite work out which one applies to you, it's best to be conservative and choose the lower figure – most of us tend to overestimate the amount of activity we do.

ACTIVITY LEVEL	ACTIVITY MULTIPLIER
Little or no exercise: (less than 3 days a week) and you have a desk job	1.2
Active: you are on your feet most of the day; for example, a stay-at-home mum with small children, or you have a desk job, but exercise at least 3 days a week	1.375
More active: you are on the move all day or you have a sedentary job but exercise vigorously 5 days a week	1.55
Highly active: you exercise vigorously 6–7 days a week, or you have a highly active job, such as construction work	1.725

Let's do some maths

If your BMR is 1,400 and you are doing little exercise, you need to do the following calculation:

$$1,400 \times 1.2 = 1,680$$

This means your body needs 1,680 calories a day to stay the same weight.

Jane Wisdom

Research suggests that those who do well in week one of their diet often do better in the long term. Why? Because they are more motivated.

HOW MANY CALORIES SHOULD YOU EAT IN A DAY TO LOSE WEIGHT?

Now you know the number of calories you need to maintain your current weight, the next step is to find out how many calories you need each day to lose weight. At Jane Plan we recommend you aim for a weight loss of between 1 and 2 pounds (between 450 and 900g) a week, which means that you will need to cut your daily calorie intake by between 500 and up to 1,000 calories a day. That's because there are about 3,500 calories in a pound of stored body fat and there are seven days in a week. So if you create a 3,500-calorie deficit by eating less you will lose a pound (450g) of body weight in a week (3,500 divided by seven equals 500). If you create a 7,000 calorie deficit you will lose 2 pounds (900g).

At Jane Plan we usually recommend a daily calorie intake of between 1,000-1,200 to help you lose weight at a rate that keeps you motivated. This works for most people, but remember, if you want to be really accurate, you'll need to do the maths as explained above.

Bear in mind that if you are much heavier, then 1,000–1,200 calories may be too little for you. If you think this might

Jane Wisdom

If you are already quite small and slim and just want to lose a little weight – perhaps for a holiday, a wedding or to get back into those skinny jeans – 1,000 calories is likely to create too great a deficit. An alternative way in these circumstances is simply to reduce your current daily calorie intake by around 15–20 per cent.

be you, it's best to go back and check your BMR to find out your ideal calorie count. (Yes, the BMR works for heavier *and* lighter people.)

I know how hard it can be to keep track of calories, so all the recipes at the back of the book are calorie counted and portion controlled, as are the Jane Plan daily menu plans, which are based on 1,000–1,200 calories a day.

MOVE MORE

A combination of diet and exercise is best for lasting weight loss. As well as cutting the calories, now is the time to dust off your trainers. I'm afraid that sustained weight loss is difficult without increased regular exercise. This doesn't mean you have to pound the pavements but you do need to move a little more. Why not keep your trainers by the front door and it will encourage you to wear them more frequently for exercise? With comfortable footwear to hand you'll walk more often and for further distances. I explain how easy it is to move more in Skinny Rule 8.

Jane Wisdom

- Don't forget, if you are a man or an active and larger woman, you may be able to eat more and still lose weight.

- As you get nearer to your weight-loss goal, or if you want to lose more than you originally decided, you may need to re-test your BMR and adjust your daily calorie count accordingly.

THE STAGES OF WEIGHT LOSS

Weight loss happens in stages, and understanding them will help you to know what to expect. Although weight loss varies from person to person, there are some common patterns. A heavier person, for example, will lose more weight in the earlier stages than a lighter person, and remember, men tend to lose weight faster than women.

Stage one As you start eating the Jane Plan way, you will be reducing your calorie, carbohydrate and salt intake, and your body will respond with rapid weight loss. It is important to recognise that some of this initial loss is water, and will not be sustained at such a rapid rate in the long term.

Stage two As the days and weeks progress, you will start to burn stored fat as well as losing water. The overall rate of weight loss, however, will slow to a steady pace. The protein element of the foods on the Jane Plan way of eating will ensure you burn fat rather than losing muscle. That's because protein helps to build muscle, and muscle helps you burn calories faster.

Stage three After a few weeks, you will stop losing water and continue to burn fat, and your weight loss should stabilise at around 1–2 pounds (450–900g) a week, which is both healthy and sustainable.

Jane Wisdom
Research has shown that teaming up with a friend can improve weight loss dramatically. It's harder to explain that 'vanishing' packet of biscuits to a friend than it is to yourself.

Jane Wisdom

As you clean up your diet and improve the quality of what you are eating as well as the quantity, the subtle flavour of fresh fruits and vegetables will really start to appeal to you more and more.

WHAT ARE PLATEAUS?

If, despite your best efforts, you reach a plateau (your weight remains the same for several weeks), you may begin to wonder why. Before you become demotivated, it is important to understand that this is quite normal – long-term results often don't show up immediately.

Hormonal changes in the week before, or the week of, your period can mean that your weight loss is not as fast as you might have expected due to fluid retention. A change in the frequency or timing of your bowel movements, and even stepping up your exercise routine, may have similar effects. Remember to always weigh in at the same time of day, preferably in the morning after you have been to the loo – the scales may show a heavier result pre-poo. Exercise can build up muscle and, as you probably know, muscle weighs more than fat. Alternatively, it could be that some old habits are creeping back, which you may not even be aware of.

The secret is not to give up and to act fast:

▶ **Check your food and exercise diary** I explain how to do this in Chapter 3. It's the best way to make sure your diet is a success. Make sure you are practising good portion control (see Skinny Rule 3, page 76) and also that you are exercising most days (see Skinny Rule 8, page 111).

▶ **Reassess your BMR** You may need to cut back on your daily calorie count.

▶ **Be strict** Go back to how you ate when you first started eating the Jane Plan way. Remember when you were worried about small points such as adding too much milk to your tea? Revisiting this feeling and sticking to the Skinny Rules – which form the backbone of the Jane Plan Diet and are explained in detail in Part Two – to the letter will help to move you off your plateau.

Jane Wisdom

Your body's calorie requirements change as you lose weight. Regularly re-testing your BMR will prevent you from plateauing, because it will help you to understand how many calories your body needs as it becomes lighter.

KNOW THAT YOU CAN SUCCEED

As you work through the book you will see that I have strategies to help you achieve success from the Jane Plan Diet, even if you slip up occasionally. Before you start, bear in mind the following:

1. Every calorie counts. If you do have a 'sneaky treat', remember that you'll need to cut back elsewhere, otherwise it will affect your weight loss.

2. Make your diet a priority. You are going to have to fit your life around it, but don't worry, the diet will soon have become so much a part of your way of life that you won't even notice it.

3. Don't have an emotional approach – be detached. See Skinny Rule 2 on page 67 for more on this.

4. If your diet doesn't go according to plan 100 per cent of the time, don't worry.

5. If you slip up, don't give up. Falling off the wagon is an inevitable part of dieting. Few people stay on track all the time. You are making big lifestyle changes. The trick is to get back on the straight and narrow as soon as you can and to focus firmly on what you have achieved so far.

6. Enjoy. Going on a diet is not a life sentence. Remember: if you enjoy something, you are much more likely to stick with it.

THE HUNGER PANGS

Feeling a little more hungry than usual is an inevitable consequence of eating less, especially at first. Think about it – your weight has accumulated over a long period of time and the chances are you have got used to eating more food than you are going to be eating the Jane Plan way.

In the Western world most of us have forgotten what real hunger feels like, because we have spent most of our life feeling full. It is not harmful and there is nothing to be scared of. Don't worry – you are not going to die of starvation. We are hard-wired to eat at the slightest twinge of hunger, but once you realise that nothing dreadful is going to happen, hunger becomes easier to cope with.

If hunger pain starts to gnaw, don't despair. It will probably take two to three days for your body to adjust to eating less. Here's how to cope:

▶ Think of a distraction: phone a friend, paint your nails, brush your teeth or go for a run.

▶ Learn to differentiate between head hunger and physical hunger. They are very different, as I explain on page 68–71.

Jane Wisdom

As you stop constantly grazing you will start to enjoy your food more, because you will feel hungry enough to savour each mouthful properly.

THE JANE PLAN DIET AT A GLANCE

Now that you know how to get started, here are the main points to help you achieve success with the Jane Plan Diet.

I recommend that you:

▶ Aim for about 1,000–1,200 calories a day depending on your weight-loss goal and your starting weight.

▶ Eat three meals a day with two healthy snacks in-between.

▶ Practise a carb curfew (no carbs after 4.00pm) in the early stages of your diet. For more on this see pages 122–3

Overleaf are ten important points to remember.

Top tips

1. **Get into the right frame of mind** Think about why you want to lose weight and what will motivate you to succeed, as well as making sure your kitchen and store-cupboard are prepared as you enter the diet zone (Chapters One, Two and Fourteen).

2. **Time it** Set a start and a finish date (pages 11–13).

3. **Record it** Keep a food diary in which you note down what, how and when you eat as well as your exercise and your weight (Chapter Three).

4. **Weigh in** Step on the scales to establish your starting weight (pages 33–5).

5. **Know your numbers** Check your BMI (body mass index) and measure your waist (pages 40–1).

6. **Count your calories** Work out your ideal daily calorie intake to achieve your goal (pages 47–50).

7. **Set your goal** Decide how much weight you want to lose (pages 39–40).

8. **Think ahead** Plan your weekly menus using recipes from the Jane Plan kitchen (Chapter Fifteen).

9. **Get going** Start to eat the Jane Plan way following the Skinny Rules to help keep you on track (Part Two).

10. **Keep it off** When you achieve your weigh-loss goal, continue to live your life the Jane Plan way (Part Four).

Part Two

■

THE SKINNY RULES

Now you know the theory behind losing weight the Jane Plan way, the next step is to put it into practice. To help you do this I'm going to share with you my Skinny Rules. Please don't be put off by the word 'rules'. It may sound like I'm wagging my finger telling you what to do, but that's not the case. I use the word 'rules' because I know that when it comes to losing weight, you have to be focused and disciplined, especially in the early stages. Remember: make losing weight a priority.

The more closely you stick to the rules, the more successful you will be in achieving long-term lasting weight loss. Having lost weight myself, I know that if you stick to the Jane Plan way of eating, you will keep it off. Think of the rules as easy-to-follow guidelines,

→

which will make your weight-loss journey a whole lot easier. What's more, they will guarantee you look and feel your best each and every day.

Practice makes perfect. We all know how to play tennis: you bounce the ball, hit it over the net and back it comes to you. But how many people actually play well? Of course, if you had a tennis coach and practised every day, you'd soon be playing like a champion. The more you do something the better at it you become.

It's the same with the Skinny Rules. If you keep practising them, in next to no time they will be second nature and you will be eating and living your life the slimmer Jane Plan way.

Chapter Five

■

SKINNY RULE 1: THINK BEFORE YOU EAT

ECOMING A CONSCIOUS EATER is perhaps the most important guiding principle of the Jane Plan way of eating. Put simply, it means that you need to think before you eat. Most of us eat unconsciously, which hampers our attempts to lose weight.

Unconscious eating occurs when you eat without paying attention to what is happening inside and outside your body. It is the act of putting food into your mouth without thinking. You miss out on the pleasure of eating – the smell of food, the enjoyment of food, its taste and texture and even the positive emotions associated with it.

Even worse than that, you don't notice when you are full. And that's why unconscious eating could be behind those unwanted pounds that keep piling on. Importantly, it can also jeopardise attempts to lose weight in the long term.

Do you think you're an unconscious eater? Don't beat yourself up about it – it's actually really hard not to be. For millions of years humans have been preconditioned to eat even when not hungry. In prehistoric times our ancestors ate for survival. Food was sparse and they ate what they could find as and when it was available. Some had 'thrifty genes', which meant that they had a predisposition to lay down fat quickly in times of abundance, a useful asset when times were lean, as they could draw on stores for energy. Their active lives (hunting, foraging, looking after children and running away from predators), and the fact that times of famine were more frequent than those of feast, meant that they rarely, if ever, got fat.

Fast forward millions of years, however, and an abundance of food, plus everyday activity being replaced by cars, escalators and labour-saving devices mean that although our bodies are still programmed to work this way, those thrifty genes work against us. We have become a society of fast food and TV dinners – disconnected from our bodies and from our food.

It is time we practised being conscious about what we are putting into our mouths and fully enjoyed our meals. Conscious eating is all about becoming aware of your physical and emotional response to food. It involves focusing on it – the smell, the taste and the texture – and increasing your enjoyment of it.

Knowing how, what, when and why you eat is the first step to achieving this.

KNOW *HOW* YOU EAT

Have you ever experienced what I call a cookie crisis? It goes like this. You're at home, watching TV or working at your desk. You're feeling a bit peckish, so you help yourself to a cookie. It's one of those yummy cookies, deliciously crumbly, yet soft in the centre – and so chocolatey.

You eat one cookie and think, Yum, that's so good; I'd like another one. So you have another one, and then another, and before you know it the packet is empty. Now you feel angry, cross with yourself for giving in. You may experience feelings of guilt or resentment.

Who knows why you started on the cookie crisis in the first place – perhaps you were bored or possibly lonely. But then the cookie eating morphed into unconscious eating as something else distracted you. It could have been the TV programme or perhaps you were busy googling and lost in another world. Whatever it was, you simply weren't aware of how you were eating.

Sounds familiar? I know I've done it, and the only way I can beat it is to think before I eat. Practising a mantra like, 'Do I *really* want this?' helps, as does making some subtle changes to your eating habits.

Simple changes add up to big results

Don't multi-task when eating It draws the focus away from the food and tempts you into mindless eating traps, like eating too much or too fast. Eating has to be a single activity – you can't do it while reading a book, surfing the web or watching TV.

Always eat sitting down If you do this you'll be less distracted and less likely to forget what you have eaten. If you eat standing up, the chances are that you will eat more of the wrong things.

Eat in one room only You wouldn't bath in the sitting room or sleep in the bathroom, so why eat anywhere but in the kitchen or the dining room? Restricting where you are 'allowed' to eat will mean you are more likely to focus on eating rather than on something else.

> *Jane Wisdom*
> Research shows that sofa scoffers eat far more. The reason?
> Eating in a slumped position can impede the speed at which
> the brain registers when you are full.

Always use a knife and fork Eating with your fingers often leads to overeating as well as bad food choices. Biscuits, crisps, bread, cakes and fries are classic finger foods – and how naughty are they? Imagine the scene: you're in a restaurant, you've ordered a super-healthy salmon and salad, your partner is having steak and chips. How often have you found yourself leaning over the table, fingers ready, to nibble on his chips?

Avoid eating on the run If you do, the chances are you won't be thinking about what you are putting into your mouth. What's more, you may easily forget you have eaten anything at all. This applies to drinks especially – you'd be amazed how many calories you can drink if you pop into Starbucks after the school run or on the way to work.

> *Jane Wisdom*
> One of those super-large cappuccinos from a high-street
> coffee shop is so calorific that it's a meal in itself.

Munch and crunch Eat slowly and chew well to give your stomach time to send a message to your brain that you have eaten something. Put your knife and fork down between each mouthful.

Go small Research shows that using smaller plates and bowls encourages smaller portions.

Jane Wisdom
Don't adopt an all-or-nothing approach. If you do succumb to a naughty nibble, stop at one and put the rest away. The secret is to stop before you do too much damage.

Always use a plate It sounds odd, but how many times do you eat straight from the packet? Avoid a cookie crisis by putting that biscuit or cake onto a plate and the rest of the packet back in the cupboard.

Jane Wisdom
Learn the balancing game – if you have had a big breakfast, go for a small lunch. Croissant at 8.00am? Then have a simple soup for lunch!

KNOW *WHAT* YOU EAT

Knowing what you eat is the next step to becoming a conscious eater. It may sound simple, but are you really aware of what you are putting into your mouth throughout the day? I am not talking about a full-blown nutritional breakdown of every single morsel, but you do need to be completely honest (with yourself) about what and how much you are eating.

How often have you treated yourself to a pizza in front of the TV, and then been surprised as you reach for the next slice to find that there are none left, or bought popcorn at the cinema and found the box empty just halfway through the film? The only way to know exactly what you are eating and how much is to keep a note of your daily food intake in your special food diary (see page 35).

KNOW *WHEN* TO EAT

Time keeping is crucial to becoming a conscious eater. To lose weight successfully the Jane Plan way you need to stick to three meals a day with two healthy snacks in between. Balancing your eating 'timetable' should stop you becoming too hungry, so you won't feel the urge to eat on the run, at your desk or anywhere else.

Jane Wisdom
When you are really hungry, it's harder to control how much you are eating. Avoid hunger – your body, like a car, needs filling up regularly to keep it firing on all cylinders.

Following the Jane Plan timetable to the letter will make it easier to combat unconscious eating. If it's not time for breakfast, lunch, dinner or a mid-morning or afternoon snack, you shouldn't be eating at all.

Breakfast Aim to eat your first meal of the day within an hour of getting up, to kick-start your digestion and boost concentration.

Mid-morning snack An 11 o'clock snack will help to keep your blood sugar levels on an even keel as well as helping to stave off pre-lunch hunger pangs. Be prepared and always have something handy from the list of snacks on pages 146–8.

Lunch Aim to eat lunch between 1.00 and 2.00pm. Too many of us leave lunch too late, which can lead to hunger and portion distortion as can skipping lunch altogether. This is not a good idea as it can lead to inappropriate food choices later in the day.

Mid-afternoon snack If you have hungry kids coming home from school demanding snacks, try to time your mid-afternoon snack with them. For those at work, time yours when colleagues may be tucking into naughty nibbles. But be a conscious eater – don't just nibble on what they are having. Have your own calorie- and portion-controlled snack to hand.

Supper Dining before 8.00pm will give your digestion time to work properly. Research suggests that late-night eaters tend to eat more and have sleep, as well as weight, problems. Also, the later you leave it the hungrier you become, which can lead to overeating.

Jane Wisdom

Shift workers often find losing weight difficult. The reason? Shift work upsets the body clock with a knock-on effect on eating patterns. The answer is to divide your waking hours into regular intervals and set your meal times accordingly, following the Jane Plan principle of breakfast, mid-morning snack, lunch, mid-afternoon snack and dinner.

KNOW *WHY* YOU EAT

Food is now available 24/7, and if you don't get to grips with why you are eating, you run the risk of eating the wrong things, in the wrong amounts, at the wrong time. See Skinny Rule 2, page 67, for more about emotional eating.

Becoming a conscious eater is a toughie! Give yourself time to learn new behaviours, and they will soon become habits. It can take several weeks of consistent practice, though, for them to kick in.

Even then, you may slip up. Remember, if you do, don't give up. The more you practise something, the better you get at it. The good news is that conscious eaters enjoy and appreciate bountiful arrays of food. What's more, they rarely have a cookie crisis.

Chapter Six

SKINNY RULE 2: CURB COMFORT EATING

OOD CAN DO MORE than just fill stomachs. When you turn to food for reasons other than hunger, it can also help to satisfy feelings – a type of eating known as emotional or comfort eating. Instead of a physical symptom of hunger initiating eating, like a rumbling tummy, an emotion such as stress, anger, boredom, low self-esteem or loneliness is the trigger. But emotional eating does not fix emotional problems and can actually make them worse. Although it may give you a quick lift, the underlying problems remain and you can end up feeling guilty for overeating and then beating yourself up for having zero willpower.

WHY DO WE COMFORT EAT?

Most of us eat for comfort from time to time, sometimes without even being aware we are doing so. People often tell me how guilty they feel, because they are 'comfort eaters', as if somehow it is their fault, but if you think about it, comfort eating is not that surprising.

As a baby, when you cried, your mother gave you milk; as you grew up, if you hurt yourself, you may have been offered sweets and treats as comfort or ice creams when you were 'good'. So from a very early age you were learning the lesson that food can make you feel better. The problem is that for some of us the idea of food being a comfort has never really gone away. You may never have learned to deal with sad or negative feelings, preferring to keep them at bay with some type of food treat.

MOOD MATTERS

According to a study carried out by Brian Wansink at Cornell University, the type of comfort food we reach for varies depending on our mood. Happy people tend to prefer foods such as pizza or steak, sad people reach for ice cream and cookies, whereas bored people tend to go for crisps. Interestingly, comfort foods can also be broken down by gender. Women tend to turn to chocolates and cookies, whereas men turn to pizza, steak and casserole; however, the one common factor is that comfort foods are usually high in calories – that's why they are such a problem.

UNDERSTAND AND DEAL WITH YOUR EMOTIONS

Learning how to deal with emotions, rather than turning to food for comfort, is a new skill that has to be learnt – otherwise losing weight for life is really hard to achieve. That's because if you eat when you are not hungry (I mean *physically* hungry), the chances are that your body does not need the calories. And if this happens too often, the extra calories get stored as fat, and the weight starts to pile on.

Jane Wisdom

Research suggests that 70 per cent of unnecessary calories are a result of comfort eating! Learning to deal with emotions and eating is crucial to weight-loss success.

Of course, using food occasionally as a pick-me-up isn't necessarily a bad thing. Food can be a genuine comfort when you are feeling under the weather. But if you find yourself heading in the direction of the fridge the minute something goes wrong, you can get stuck in an unhealthy cycle of overeating without ever addressing the real problem that caused you to feel the need to eat in the first place.

Learning to recognise what makes you eat like this is the way to break free from food cravings and change the habits that may have ruined your diet attempts in the past.

The first step is to identify the difference between physical hunger and emotional hunger.

Physical hunger is:

▶ Gradual. Your stomach may gurgle or rumble.

▶ Open to options. When you eat because you are hungry, you are happy with a wide variety of food choices rather than craving a specific food, such as chocolate.

▶ Uncomfortable. You may get a slight headache.

▶ Felt in the stomach. You feel an emptiness in the pit of your stomach.

▶ Not accompanied by guilt afterwards.

And it:

▶ Makes you feel tired and irritable.

▶ Stops when you are full.

Emotional hunger:

▶ Urges you to eat NOW.

▶ Is often linked with a bad day: a child in trouble, a row with your partner, something going wrong at work.

▶ Often takes the form of a craving for a particular food or drink, such as chocolate, biscuits, cakes, wine.

▶ Is absentminded. You may not notice how much you have eaten or you simply keep eating, even when you are full.

▶ Makes you feel guilty afterwards.

Once you have learnt the difference between emotional and physical hunger, the next step is to identify what makes you reach for the comfort of food.

Common triggers include:

▶ Feeling empty, low or lonely

▶ Tiredness and fatigue

▶ PMT or menopausal problems

▶ Grief

- ▶ Stress

- ▶ Boredom

- ▶ Low self-esteem

- ▶ An urge to celebrate

- ▶ A really bad day/experience

Once you have identified your personal triggers, you need to find another way of managing these feelings, which doesn't involve reaching for the biscuit tin.

Recognise what triggers your comfort eating, so don't skip filling in that column in your food diary.

COPING TACTICS

If you are feeling lonely and depressed, try phoning a close friend or family member who usually makes you feel better. Make a date to go to a film or see an exhibition. Doing something productive will make you feel better!

If you are tired, have a lovely hot bath, light a scented candle or take a quick nap.

If you are stressed, take up meditation or some sort of relaxation exercise such as yoga. Occupying your hands with knitting or sewing can also be therapeutic.

If you are sad, do something for yourself such as going for an aromatherapy massage. Alternatively, getting out of the house and exercising will release endorphins – the body's natural feel-good hormones that enhance mood.

If you are bored, engross yourself in a good book, do some gardening or DIY, or start researching your next holiday. Research suggests that even planning a trip can boost mood.

If you're in the mood to celebrate, take some photos of what's making you so happy – the party, your friends, or whatever it is. Concentrating on recording the moment will keep you away from the food.

Jane Wisdom

Sometimes you just need to stay with the feeling. Stop trying to escape it. Don't do anything. Just observe it quietly and calmly without judgement. The chances are that if you do this it will go away. This is the principle behind mindfulness.

LET GO OF GUILT

When it comes to comfort eating, all too often willpower, self-discipline and good intentions fall by the wayside. You start to eat chocolate, cheese, biscuits and bread, and the downward spiral begins. You feel guilty. You feel miserable, so what do you do? STOP? No – actually, you end up eating not just a nibble but an entire packet.

You justify it, 'I've had a terrible day. I'm just having a treat. The diet can start again tomorrow.' Sounds familiar? Don't feel guilty – remember that comfort eating is a learned behaviour and by practising some of the techniques above you can unlearn it!

STAND UP TO CRAVINGS

A food craving – a powerful urge to eat a particular type of food – is a typical response to emotional eating. It can be so all-consuming that you can think of nothing else until you have satisfied it. But the truth is you have more control of your cravings than you think. The secret is to give a craving some time – to delay eating for a few minutes.

The ten-minute trick As soon as you feel yourself being swept along by a craving, ask yourself, 'Do I need this or do I just want this?' Wait for ten minutes and ask yourself the same question again. A food craving usually builds up to a peak before slowly drifting away again.

The toothpaste trick If the craving is still there after ten minutes, try brushing your teeth, drinking a large glass of water or chewing a piece of gum – it might just do the trick.

Jane Wisdom
Always carry toothpaste in your bag, and keep a toothbrush in the nearest loo – that way you'll see it every time you pop in, and it will remind you to brush your teeth.

If the craving simply won't go away, ask yourself, 'How will I feel if I choose to eat? How will I feel if I don't?' If you decide to give in, have a small portion, put it on a plate and sit down to eat it as far away from the fridge or cupboard as possible.

DON'T BE AN ALL-OR-NOTHING THINKER

A really desperate cookie crisis can lead to all-or-nothing thinking, not to mention dramatic language, such as, 'It's a disaster!', 'I hate myself!', 'What's the point of going on?', 'I am so hopeless!', 'I've no self-control!' Just because you have had one lapse does not mean you have to continue or that your diet has gone out the window. One diet lapse doesn't make you a failure.

Although biscuits are banned in the Jane Plan way of eating, tell yourself that it's OK to have one occasionally. But don't have one too often; sugar can be addictive, but the good news is that if you cut it out the chances are you will soon lose the taste for it. Instead of thinking of yourself as a failure when you give way to a craving, remind yourself that tomorrow is another day and that you can get back on track. Be realistic – slip-ups do happen, but you can also overcome and learn from them.

Jane Wisdom
Jane Plan allows yummy treats in the right quantity at the right time.

Jane Wisdom
Whether it reduces your calorie intake by 200 calories a day or whether it stops you bingeing, you need to curb comfort eating to lose weight for life.

WHAT YOUR CRAVINGS SAY ABOUT YOU

If you crave ...	You could be ...	Try
Salty foods	Stressed and angry	Crunching on some celery. Taking up meditation or yoga
Red meat	Tired and lethargic	A lean cut of steak on a bed of beans
Cheese/pizza	Anxious and insecure, in need of some comfort	A handful of walnuts, wild salmon, mixed seeds
Sweets	Low in blood sugar and in need of a hug	Fruit such as a handful of berries
Bread, pasta, rice (carbs)	Stressed and low in energy	An oatcake, wholemeal tabbouleh or couscous
Coffee	In need of a pick-me-up	Biting an apple. It will give you more energy than a shot of caffeine

Chapter Seven

■

SKINNY RULE 3: BEAT PORTION DISTORTION

I **AM OFTEN ASKED** if there is one thing you can do that would make a real difference to weight loss. Portion control is my answer. At Jane Plan I suggest you cut your portions by about a third. Why? You may already be eating very healthily, but are eating just a little bit too much. Increasing your portions even by a modest amount can, over time, cause weight gain.

No matter how healthy your diet, if your portions are too large, and you're taking in more energy than you are expending, you'll put on weight. But at Jane Plan we are only too aware of how hard it can be to control your portions. The reason? Over the past two decades portion sizes have grown bigger and bigger, which means your perception of what constitutes the right-sized portion may have become distorted.

Many restaurants now serve portions that are far larger than your body needs. And that's not all. Studies show that when presented with more food than you need, most of us eat it without even giving it a second thought. They also show, however, that if presented with less you still feel satisfied, as an intriguing study carried out at Penn State University in the US shows.

In the experiment, researchers gave one group of participants a standard serving of pasta, while another group was given a serving that was half as big again. Afterwards they asked the participants how satisfied they felt after eating. Amazingly, people in both groups said the portions they had been served were just right for their needs. Those served the larger portion had eaten nearly all of it, however, adding an extra 172 calories to their meal. The lesson is clear: if you are watching your weight, smaller portions can be just as satisfying as the larger ones you may be used to.

It's the same story in supermarkets and shops. Food is now sold in much larger packets, and research shows that the bigger the packet – be it spaghetti in the kitchen or cereal on the table – the more you tend to serve yourself. And this can be as much as 30 per cent more, say the experts.

The fact is you have become so used to seeing large portions that if you are served smaller ones you imagine that you have been short-changed. And that doesn't just apply to eating out; people also serve themselves whopping portions at home. These big portions have become the norm.

DID YOU KNOW?

A study by the Food Standards Agency found that ready-meal portions have grown significantly in the last few years; for example, a shop-bought beef lasagne averaged around 250g in 1999 but by 2008 had grown to 500g.

BECOME PORTION AWARE

Whether you want to lose weight or maintain your current weight loss the only way to survive these trends is to become more portion aware; however, as most people tend to under-estimate how many calories they are eating from day to day, this can be difficult. Do you really know, for example, what the recommended serving of uncooked porridge oats of 40g looks like? (It's equivalent to one 57 × 25mm ramekin.) Most people tend to pour much more into their breakfast cereal bowl, which can add extra calories and scupper the best-laid diet goals. So what is the answer?

Measuring and weighing everything you put into your mouth is time-consuming and extremely tedious. To make things simpler, I suggest you use a handful as your guideline and familiar objects such as your iPhone or a tennis ball as a rough guide against which to measure your portions. The secret is to learn to become visually aware of what constitutes a portion so that you can see at a glance whether it's too much or 'just right'.

Jane Wisdom

Many people are surprised when they realise what a typical portion size should look like. If you're used to piling your plate high with pasta or filling your bowl to the brim with cereal, it can come as quite a shock, but once you cut down, you'll soon get used to eating less.

WHAT'S IN A PORTION?

Study the chart below to help you become more visually aware of portion size.

One portion of:	Equals the size of:
Cereal or uncooked porridge	Ramekin dish (57 × 25mm)
Rice or pasta, uncooked	Tennis ball
Lean meat	iPhone
Fish	Cheque book
Hard cheese	Small matchbox
Vegetables	1 handful
Salad	Cereal bowl
Fruit	1 handful
Pulses, uncooked	3 heaped tablespoons
Soup	Cereal bowl or a medium-sized mug
Butter or olive oil	Tip of your thumb
Potato	Small computer mouse such as an Apple
Milk – when adding to tea or coffee	More than a splash is a waste (max. 2cm in the cup)
Pancake – treat days only	CD
Crisps – treat days only	Cupped handful
Nuts	These vary in calories so you have to count them out*

*See my Skinny Snacks, Mini Mouthfuls and Harmless Handfuls on page 146.

HOW TO WISE UP TO PORTIONS

Making small tweaks to the size of your portions can make a big positive difference to your calorie intake and won't leave you feeling hungry.

At home

Avoid eating from containers, mixing bowls or saucepans Seeing food on a plate or in a bowl gives you a better idea of portion size. Nibbling while cooking is a hard one to break, but follow this tip and you will break the habit for life.

Reduce plate size In a study carried out at Cornell University, reducing plate size from 30cm to 25cm led to 22 per cent fewer calories being consumed. Also, a small plate full of food is much less disheartening than a large plate that's half empty.

Plate up in the kitchen rather than serving at the table – it will stop you thinking you want more.

Put away or freeze leftovers as soon as you can, to reduce the risk of going back for seconds.

Serve yourself slightly less than you think you will eat.

Eat slowly It takes twenty minutes for your brain to register that you are full, so taking your time allows your brain to catch up with the signals coming from your digestive system.

Never eat out of a bag or packet Listen up, biscuit bunnies, this tip will save you from a cookie crisis.

If you must have seconds, choose vegetables.

Drink a large glass of water before every meal – it will make you feel full.

In the shops

Buy portion-divided foods. You are less likely to get through several individual servings in one go, whereas it can be easy to get through a whole packet.

If buying ready meals, choose calorie-controlled options.

Avoid extra-value foods or meal deals.

Read labels carefully. Packaged foods usually show portion or serving information on the nutritional fact box, but beware: unless you look carefully, it is easy to think the servings are for the whole packet while in fact they may be for just half.

If you can't stop yourself eating ice cream out of the tub, buy individual-sized servings.

Avoid multi-buys – you can end up eating more.

Jane Wisdom

- Repack big boxes of cereal and packets of spaghetti into smaller containers. You'll serve yourself less from a smaller container.

- Watch out for healthy food labels – just because they say they are healthy does not give you the green light to eat more. They can still be high in calories.

In restaurants

Restaurant portions can be large, and in pub restaurants they are sometimes even larger. Eat slowly, and as soon as you start to feel full, stop and ask for a take-home bag.

Ask for sauces and dressings to be put on the side then use a teaspoon to serve them.

In coffee shops, go for a basic filter coffee – a standard size used to be around 200ml (45 calories with milk and sugar) but is now around 354ml.

If a pizza is more than 25cm across, share it – US research suggests an average pizza serving has a massive 850 calories today compared with 500 calories 20 years ago.

Have a starter and soup or salad instead of a main course.

If you can't go without pudding, ask someone to share it with you.

Choose from the children's menu Or simply ask for a small portion.

Jane Wisdom
The best part of pudding is often the first two bites so why not share if you must have one.

Chapter Eight

■

SKINNY RULE 4: SAY NO TO NAUGHTY NIBBLING

TIME AFTER TIME, when I ask women why they think losing weight is such a struggle, they reply, 'I just eat all day', 'I can't stop snacking', 'I'm always nibbling at something' or 'I see food and just have to eat it!' (Interestingly, when I ask men the same question, they usually cite portion size as their major downfall.)

Whether you call it snacking, grazing or naughty nibbling, constantly eating tiny amounts is a common downfall. As people graze their way through the day they are mindlessly taking in calories they don't need and food they often forget they have even eaten.

If you never sit down to a meal or can't walk past a plate of biscuits without picking one up, the chances are you are in the ranks of the naughty nibblers – but rest assured, you are not alone.

Research shows that one in ten of us spends up to £35 a week on sweet snacks and drinks – that's almost £2,000 a year or £7 every weekday. It's hardly surprising we're in the middle of an obesity epidemic.

WHY DO WE SNACK SO OFTEN?

Endless working hours, changing work patterns and long commutes have turned us into a nation of nibblers, according to research, which has found that Britons nibble or snack more than people in any other country in Europe.

The conflicting advice from the media over the years about how we should eat is another reason. 'Little and often' is the buzzword of the moment, but what does this phrase actually mean? It's usually touted as a way of keeping blood sugar levels on an even keel and is meant to discourage us from overeating unhealthy food. Eating little and often will give you a constant supply of energy; if you leave long gaps between eating you risk your blood sugar levels dropping and then eating too much to compensate. The problem is that some of us seem to ignore the 'little' and only hear the 'eat often'.

As a result, we're snacking more than ever before and often on unhealthy foods, which is ruining our ability to control our weight. And even if we do go for so-called 'healthy' snacks, such as nuts and dried fruit, many of us seem to think this gives us the green light to snack as much as we like, forgetting that even healthy snacks can be laden with calories, fat or sugar. Recently, the government has encouraged food producers to reduce the saturated fat element in processed foods in an attempt to make them 'healthier', but it's very important to realise that processed foods, especially cakes, biscuits, pies, snacks, bars, chocolate (unless made with a high percentage of cocoa solids) are never healthy, regardless of what the labels might say, and that eating them only makes you crave more of those types of foods, leading to weight gain.

The Jane Plan way of eating does not encourage mindless grazing or snacking, and naughty nibbling doesn't feature either! But it does allow you two healthy, wisely chosen, portion-controlled snacks every day. Just two – no more! That way you will keep hunger at bay and you won't fall into the portion-distortion trap at meals.

ALL ABOUT PROTEIN

It's widely accepted now that some protein should feature in every meal, and this includes snacks. Why? Because protein makes you feel fuller for longer; however, when it comes to snacks, the problem is that often protein is not very portable. And most of us have neither the luxury nor the time to be able to sit down at the kitchen table mid-morning or mid-afternoon to eat a perfectly balanced snack.

How hard is it to add protein to a mid-morning or afternoon snack if you are working in an office, on the school run or driving in the car? Hummus can be very messy to eat! Ham in the handbag? Not for me! But that doesn't mean you have to resort to the biscuit tin.

Jane Plan is all about making weight loss easy – so don't beat yourself up if you read in a magazine or newspaper that you should have protein with every meal (including snacks) – it won't ruin your diet if you don't. And remember, protein contains exactly the same amount of calories as carbs! The secret is to choose a snack that works for you.

Jane Wisdom

Eat the Jane Plan way and your two snacks a day won't derail your diet or be unhealthy as long as you choose wisely.

SUPER-SNACKS

A well-planned, nutritious nibble, such as a few sticks of carrot, celery or red, yellow or green pepper slices with some low-fat hummus, can help you stay energised, boost your day's nutrients and help prevent overeating at meal times. But if you can't do the hummus, then don't worry, the crudités alone make a fabulous snack.

And that's not all. Concentration levels often fall between meals when blood sugar levels drop. A judiciously chosen snack, such as an oatcake with a dollop of low-fat cottage cheese or a couple of portions of sushi, can help sharpen your brain and contribute to your daily nutritional intake. But again, if you can't find a way to include the cottage cheese, an apple will do the trick.

Get the timing right

The secret is it must be the right snack, at the right time in the right quantity. Two snacks a day: the first one two to three hours after breakfast will help to keep you energised and curb pre-lunch hunger pangs; and another around 3.00–4.00pm will help avoid that familiar mid-afternoon slump.

Jane Wisdom
Remember: snacks are not calorie-free. Yes, they do
contribute to your overall calorie count for the day.

Stress-free skinny snacks

Living life and losing weight the Jane Plan way is all about
things that are easy and doable, including snacking habits. You
need to make sure you have easy nibbles to hand so that you
can get them out at your specified snack time.

If you don't have time to plan or even think, try:

▶ Fruit, such as two plums, two easy-peel satsumas, a medium
banana (no more than two a week, though, as they are high
in sugar), one good-sized apple.

▶ Nuts – but watch your portion control here. Although packed
with protein, nuts are high in fat and are very moreish. Count
out nine almonds or two walnuts or Brazil nuts.

▶ A packet of miso soup.

▶ Two rice cakes or oatcakes.

If you have a fridge at work or you are at home during the day, try:

▶ A small piece of cheese – about the same size as your thumb.

▶ Babybel cheese.

▶ Individual pot of low-fat yogurt.

▶ A handful of berries such as strawberries or blueberries.

If you have more time on your hands, try:

▶ One to two handfuls of crudités, such as carrots, celery, pepper, radishes or mangetouts. (Cut them up the night before to take with you to work the next day.)

▶ Two Ryvitas or crispbreads with 1 tablespoonful of hummus or cottage cheese.

▶ A handful of small olives.

▶ A hard-boiled egg.

▶ A handful of edamame beans.

▶ A handful of cut fruit, such as an orange, wedge of watermelon, slice of pineapple, half a mango or half a grapefruit.

▶ Sushi.

(See Chapter sixteen for more ideas.)

ARE YOU A NAUGHTY NIBBLER?

Study the questions below. If you answer yes to any, it is time to follow the advice to stop that naughty nibbling. If you don't, you will soon start to gain weight often without even realising it.

1. Do you graze throughout the day?
Make sure there are no visible snacks wherever you are! Remember: you eat with your eyes. Out of sight, out of mind!

2. Are you consistently nibbling at your desk or in meetings? Make your office space a food-free zone. Ask for fresh fruit and water at meetings – and ask colleagues not to bring in the biscuits and coffee.

3. Are you a fridge forager?
   Do you find it hard to pass the fridge without sneaking a look inside? Stick goal alerts on the fridge door.

4. Is your handbag full of naughty nibbles?
   Make your handbag a sacred place for keys, money and makeup only. Clear out any crumbs from the bottom NOW.

5. Do you crunch away in the car?
   Ban eating in the car – and that applies to the children too. Crumbs under car seats are a nightmare to clean up.

6. Do you stop and shop for snacks while out and about?
   Make sure you don't have any small change in your pockets – that way you won't be able to pay for any naughty nibbles.

7. Do you nibble on trains and buses?
   People eating on the train can be a horrid sight. Imagine how you will look munching away. What will other people think? Do you want to become that person? Eating on the move – except of course on long-distance plane, boat, train or car journeys – is a firm no-no the Jane Plan way.

8. If you have children, do you suffer from the five o'clock fish-finger moment?
   At children's teatime, put a plate of crudités in the middle of the table and nibble from that instead. Remember: children learn from example – if you can't stop nibbling from their plates for yourself, at least stop for them.

9. Do you eat while feeding the baby? One spoon for baby, one spoon for you?
   It might make time pass faster, but it may also stop you ever getting back to your pre-pregnancy weight.

10. Do you eat off your partner's plate?
Keep your hands to yourself and play footsie instead.

11. Do you automatically load the toaster when boiling the kettle?
Put the toaster away in the cupboard – at least for the first few weeks of your new Jane Plan lifestyle.

12. Do you find it hard to resist a muffin when ordering a mid-morning cappuccino?
Start by switching that cappuccino to a herbal tea, and stop kidding yourself that you need that muffin. Ask yourself, 'Do I really need to use up so many calories of my daily allowance at 11.00am?'

13. Are you a biscuit-tin bunny? Do you always have to have a biscuit with a cup of tea?
Ban the biscuit tin. A packet of biscuits in the house is hard to resist – and don't think you will stick to just one!

14. Do you lick the bowl after baking?
Remember the rule – never eat while standing up. Put the bowl away in the dishwasher as soon as you can.

15. Do you taste as you cook?
If you are not careful, you can end up consuming the calorie equivalent of a whole meal while cooking, so why even contemplate it? Use a teaspoon, not a tablespoon, to sample your cooking. One teaspoon is enough to tell if you need to adjust the seasoning.

16. Do you eat from the shopping trolley?
Never shop while hungry. If you do slip up on the treats while shopping, put them away in an opaque box and hide them behind something healthier in the cupboard.

ARE YOU A NIGHT-TIME NIBBLER?

Over the years, many people have told me that their weakest moment is at night. 'I do so well all day, but come the evening, it all falls apart,' is a familiar moan. This may be because they are more relaxed, their time is less structured or because once they have created a pattern of eating, they find it hard to break.

If this sounds familiar, it's time to change your evening routine.

▶ If you come home from work and munch your way through the contents of the fridge before even taking off your jacket, don't go into the kitchen. Make the bedroom the first room you enter, and change your clothes before going into the kitchen.

▶ If you tend to snack in front of the TV, make sure you eat dinner before you tune in.

▶ If you start to nibble late at night, simply going to bed earlier can help.

Chapter Nine

■

SKINNY RULE 5:
BEWARE
THE DIET DESTROYERS

I'S HARD ENOUGH to lose weight alone, but it's harder still
if friends and family aren't supportive or, worse still, start
to scupper your efforts to stay slim. The current television
trend for cookery programmes doesn't help much either, nor
do the glowing restaurant reviews in the Sunday supplements,
not to mention the endless pages of tempting recipes in the
latest cookery books and magazines.

Food, after all, is all about giving and sharing. It's what you
do with your families and friends – both out of necessity and
to celebrate special occasions. You sit down to eat with one
another, go out to restaurants together, compare recipes and
follow blogs. And if you're a foodie, the chances are you also
avidly read cookery books and the recipe pages are often the
first you turn to in magazines and newspapers.

You are bombarded on all sides by TV chefs and reality
cooking shows. Gorgeous images of food look down on you

from billboards. Food is everywhere, and it is important that you don't underestimate the knock-on effect this can have on what and how you eat.

Closer to home, you may be the family meal provider, which can make it difficult to establish different eating patterns from your family. You may not want to appear the odd one out. And then there are those well-meaning – or perhaps not so well-meaning – friends or family members.

All need not be lost. There are ways to turn your back on the diet saboteurs as well as breaking down any barriers that may be standing between you and the Jane Plan way of eating.

MEDIA POWER

The effects of TV chefs and cooking programmes, volumes of recipe books and endless food blogs, which have become integral to 21st-century living, are difficult to combat and, let's face it, are not going to go away. The only way to cope is to accept them for what they are. Learn to live with them. Become more conscious and aware of their influence on your eating habits, and you will be half-way there.

▶ Not all recipe cards and recipes are necessarily high in calories, so study them carefully and pick out the ones with the lower count.

▶ Avoid leafing through the dessert section in cookery books and focus on salads instead.

▶ Look for food blogs that promote healthy eating, such as smarterfitter.com – there are loads of others or switch to exercise or fashion blogs such as Net-a-Porter.

▶ Avert your eyes when passing cafés and enticing food-shop windows. Creating a mantra can help; for example, at the first sign of a craving, call to mind the old favourite 'a moment on the lips is a lifetime on the hips'.

▶ Swap food magazines for *Vogue* or *Glamour* or sports or hobby mags. Becoming voyeuristic about stilettos or the latest fitness gear rather than cream cakes is the way to go.

▶ If you come across a gorgeous recipe, of course, you must try it – apply the Jane Plan principles of portion control and you should be OK. Consider a once-a-week splurge night – use it as an opportunity to recreate some of the delights you have been reading about. But always with an eye on portion control.

FAMILY PRESSURE

As a mum of three I am only too aware of the constant pressure (and pleasure) in cooking and providing food for the family. Sharing at the table, after all, is the crux of family life, but at the same time it is what makes it so hard to maintain that svelte pre-children figure as well as the yummy-mummy image that is expected of us. Teenage sons and husbands, for example, require a lot more pasta and potatoes than you, and these foods can be hard to resist when they are there on the table.

The answer is to put some protective strategies in place. Encouraging the family to eat the types of food you like is a good place to start. It's good for them too! You can always have an extra bowl of jacket potatoes, rice or pasta ready to fill them up as long as you steer clear yourself.

If you are nervous about watching your calories in front of the children, the best thing is not to mention what you are doing and carry on as normal. If they start to make comments, tell them you are trying to eat more healthily rather than saying you are on a diet.

Jane Wisdom

Ask your partner not to offer you seconds – that way you avoid having to say 'no thanks' in public.

WEEKEND WISDOM

Sunday lunch can be tricky when you are watching your weight. Here's how to get through it while still sticking to the Jane Plan way to eat.

► Plate up food rather than putting help-yourself bowls on the table. That way you avoid everyone staring or, worse still, making sarcastic remarks when you pass on the roasties or Yorkshire pud.

► Always buy lean cuts of meat, and cut off any visible fat and remove skin – remember your portion should be the size of the palm of your hand. *No bigger now*!

► Serve plenty of interesting veggies – carrots and broccoli for the children, *plus* asparagus and courgettes for you. Variety is the spice of life.

► Grilled veg, such as courgettes or aubergines, make the meal more interesting and are a great alternative to lashings of fattening gravy.

→

▶ Fresh fruit or iced sorbets are far better choices than the staple Sunday apple crumble.

Saturday lunch or dinner with the kids can be just as tough.

▶ If serving pasta, keep it for the children and serve yourself the sauce on a pile of green veg, such as beans, mangetouts or courgettes. Or invest in one of those clever spiral slicers that will make courgette or carrot 'spaghetti' – or see the recipe for Courgette Spaghetti on page 237. (Remember: tomato-based sauces are always better than cream. To add a creamy touch use crème fraîche.)

▶ Everyone loves pizza, and two or three slices of the lower-cal versions, such as classic Margarita, are OK as an occasional treat. Don't be tempted, though, by the dough balls and dressings.

▶ Make sure you have a big bowl of salad in the middle of the table. You can serve yourself a mountain as well as encouraging everyone else to have some too.

▶ Weekend meals are a wonderful opportunity to introduce the children to more interesting foods that they may not have tried before. Most love simple grilled salmon or baked chicken – it doesn't always have to be pizza and pasta.

AVOID THE DIET RIVALS

There is no escaping the fact that some women are out to sabotage their friends' diet attempts – they are often not as supportive as they could be. There are diet saboteurs everywhere. They will be offering you crisps and nibbles before dinner, making comments about how little you have on your plate, casting suspicious glances as you say no to pud – and telling you how wonderful you look and that you don't need to lose any weight!

So why do they do this? 'When you choose to look after yourself, improve or lose weight, other people feel threatened; it's as though they see it as a personal rebuke or affront to themselves,' explains Carole Ann Rice, life coach and author of The Real Coaching Company. She suggests:

> When you hang out with other people who may have weight issues you can enjoy a 'we're in it together' sort of camaraderie and share excuses. But when you decide to break out and lose weight and get into shape it throws their own issues into sharp relief and makes them feel bad so they want to drag you back to their negative way of thinking. If friends continue to sabotage you then seek others who understand your goal and desire to look and feel better and let them cheerlead you to success.

STAND FIRM

The secret is to focus firmly on your goals. Think about the Hollywood stars – do you think they stop their diet because someone offers them a sausage roll? If they have a red-carpet moment coming up, you can bet they are focused, still out socialising, but definitely ignoring their friends (or should we call them diet rivals?).

Remember: you are doing this for yourself and no one else, and there is no need to justify your actions or rationale to anyone. In fact, there is no need to even tell anyone what you are doing – and studies show that people who keep schtum about their diet end up doing better than those who shout about it from the rooftops.

Here's how to answer back to catty comments/back-handers:

▶ 'You haven't got much on your plate.'
You: 'It's fine, I can always come back for more.'

▶ 'Aren't you going to have pudding?'
You: 'I'm not really a pudding person, but I wouldn't mind some fruit. Have you got any?'

▶ 'You've lost loads of weight; are you OK?'
You: 'Yes, I'm fine, thanks. I'm eating the Jane Plan way and just feel so much better.'

▶ 'Don't you like potatoes then?'
You: 'Yes I do, but I'm not that hungry this lunchtime as I had a late breakfast.'

▶ 'Are you on a diet?'
You: 'No, not exactly. I'm learning to eat the Jane Plan way.'

▶ 'You are slim enough already – you don't need to lose weight.'
You: 'That's kind of you to say, but I'm a great believer in nipping excess pounds in the bud.'

Chapter Ten

SKINNY RULE 6: STOP DRINKING YOUR CALORIES

THE LATEST GOVERNMENT statistics show that behind the closed doors of many homes, alcohol consumption has reached an all-time high. And, unlike in the past, women are now the biggest culprits.

Almost one in five women drinks to excess – and the number drinking more than the recommended maximum number of units (14 a week for a woman) has grown by a fifth over the past decade, according to figures released by the Office for National Statistics. By contrast, men's drinking habits have remained constant over the past ten years. (The recommended maximum number of units for a man is 21.)

Ladies, we lead tough, stressful lives, and I know that even pouring a drop of wine into a glass can instil a feeling of calm, but if you're trying to lose weight the Jane Plan way, alcohol is a definite no-no – certainly in the first two weeks or so.

The reason? Not only is alcohol high in calories (about 7 calories per gram, almost as high as fat), but it also has little nutritional value. What's more, it can add unwanted pounds, push up blood pressure, damage your liver as well as increasing the risk of some cancers, including breast cancer. So cutting back on alcohol isn't just good for your waistline, it's good for your health too.

And of course, after a couple of drinks, you are more likely to lose your 'diet' resolve. As the old saying goes, 'Willpower is soluble in alcohol.' That said, I do know how hard it can be to give up that evening glass of wine for good, so if you're really struggling, try to give up completely during your first week, then have a re-think to see if you can bear another wine-free week. Keep repeating this exercise, remembering that it takes 28 days to break a habit. After a month re-introduce wine at weekends, but no more than two glasses on two nights. Pour your wine into a tall, thin glass, and make sure you always take three sips of water for every sip of wine to keep yourself fully hydrated.

Jane Wisdom
Always buy the best-quality wine you can afford, and savour every sip. You will drink less, and the more expensive the wine the less you will be tempted to just glug it down without thinking.

Jane Wisdom
Don't be a 'sofa slurper': sipping on the sofa in front of the TV is a no-no. It increases the risk of you drinking more – often without you even realising.

RESIST TEMPTATION

I also know how tricky some moments can be when you would just kill for a glass of wine; for example, straight after work; when the children go to bed; or while cooking the dinner. The secret is to put some coping strategies in place to stop you reaching for the bottle.

The office-to-the-wine-bar moment

It's easy to get into the habit of rushing from the office to the wine bar in an attempt to relax after the pressures of the day, but the truth is a glass or two of wine will increase stress levels as well as expanding your waistline.

> ### Jane Wisdom
> Adopt another habit such as going to the gym or running. If it's company you're after, go to a film after work with a friend or for a browse around the shops on your way home.

The wine-o'clock moment

Mums, you know this only too well. As soon as the kids hit the pillow all you want is a glass of wine.

> ### Jane Wisdom
> Don't keep chilled wine in the fridge. Pour yourself some fizzy mineral water or a slim-line tonic, add a slice of lemon or lime and some crushed ice. Then sit down and savour it.

The chop-chop-chop-sip-sip-sip moment

You open the bottle as you're cooking supper, but before you know it you have quaffed half of it before you've even sat down at the table.

> *Jane Wisdom*
>
> Keep the bottle unopened until dinner is ready and listen to music as you cook – it will help to fill the void the glass of wine has left.

The secret-drinking moment

You nip into kitchen after your dinner guests have gone and carry on drinking.

> *Jane Wisdom*
>
> Stop kidding yourself that you deserve it. All you are doing is adding another 180 calories to your daily count, not to mention increasing the risk of a nasty hangover. Think of wine as a treat to be enjoyed with family and friends.

Chapter Eleven

■

SKINNY RULE 7:
WISE UP TO EATING OUT

BEING A CONSCIOUS EATER can be more of a challenge when you go out to eat, but as long as you are mindful of the menu and follow the Skinny Rules on portion control, there is no reason why it should damage your waistline. Look at what is on your plate at all times and ask yourself, 'Do I really want this?'

AT THE BUFFET

Buffets can be full of temptation. Remember: the biggest pleasure is in meeting and talking with others rather than the food.

▶ Visit the buffet table once, and then stand as far away from it as you can.

▶ Avoid high-fat foods and stick to fresh and green salad items.

▶ Practise portion control – make sure the porcelain of the plate is always visible.

SUMMER BARBECUES

The wafting smell of food cooking on the barbecue on long sunny evenings can be irresistible. Try to stick with grilled fish, lean meat and vegetables, but if you must have a burger or steak use the following strategies:

▶ No buns or garlic bread.

▶ Avoid the crisps and nibbles, which are often in full flow, as barbecue food is invariably late.

▶ Go for salads and avoid potatoes.

▶ Choose chicken and fish options – if you can't say no to red meat, choose one type and stick to one portion. Just because it's a barbecue it doesn't mean you have to have sausages *and* burgers *and* steak – you wouldn't pile your plate like this at any other occasion.

DRINKS PARTIES

The downfall of many a dieter, but as with buffets the secret is to focus on the people rather than the drinks tray.

▶ Take a leaf out of the top models' book: keep your champagne or wine glass full at all times (that means sipping it very occasionally) – that way it won't get topped up.

▶ Give the canapés a miss. If you can't, restrict yourself to three over the evening. Make sure you go for the ones you really like and you won't feel deprived.

▶ Earn some brownie points – offer to drive!

BUSINESS MEETINGS

Breakfast and working lunches can be challenging. As the host, you may feel obliged to indulge to ensure your clients and colleagues feel relaxed, and as a guest, you may want to be seen to be enjoying the corporate hospitality.

What's more, it can be difficult to make the right choices when faced with plates of hot croissants or calorie-laden sandwiches, but following some Jane Plan conscious-eating strategies should help to keep you on the right track.

The breakfast meeting

If you have a breakfast meeting to attend, eat a Jane Plan breakfast (see page 150) before you go, and drink coffee or tea at the meeting – avoid high-calorie juices.

If it would be rude to refuse food, choose fresh fruit and yoghurt. Don't be tempted by mini croissants and muffins. They are loaded with sugar and fat and can lead to a sharp rise followed by a dip in blood sugar levels, leaving you feeling hungry later in the morning.

A working lunch

When faced with boardroom sandwiches:

▶ Restrict yourself to half a sandwich. Pick ones made with brown or granary bread and filled with lean meat such as chicken or, even better, salmon or cottage cheese. Don't eat the crusts.

▶ Avoid anything with mayonnaise.

▶ Alternatively, tell your colleagues that you are following a wheat-free diet (it's easier than saying you're trying to lose weight – probably not something you want to discuss at a business meeting anyway).

▶ Eat the fillings only.

If lunching in a restaurant:

▶ Order a simple green salad with dressing on the side, or order one course only.

▶ Say no to the bread basket.

▶ Tell your friends and colleagues you have already had a working breakfast or are going out to dinner in the evening. That way they won't expect you to eat so much.

▶ Set yourself a deadline to leave (before dessert) and say you are in a rush, which is why you can't eat too much.

▶ Drink plenty of water.

▶ Check out the menu in advance and suggest a place that serves small portions and healthy food.

▶ Avoid heavy, rich food options. They may look tempting but chances are they are high in calories and may trigger an afternoon slump.

▶ Go for sushi or, even better, sashimi whenever you can. It is the perfect low-calorie lunch provided you steer clear of the sticky rice.

Jane Wisdom

Don't feel you have to finish everything on your plate. Leaving a little something behind is a sure sign you've become a conscious eater.

Dining out

Dining out in restaurants plays a bigger part in 21st-century life than ever before, so learning to be aware of what you put on your dinner plate has never been so important.

▶ Don't be shy about choosing a simple salad, a starter only, or a plate of vegetables. Tell your friends you have had a big lunch and are not that hungry.

▶ Choose simply cooked plain food and avoid sauces.

▶ Ask the waiter to explain how the dishes are cooked and, if necessary, ask him to make some tweaks, such as no butter on the grilled fish, and salad dressings and sauces on the side.

▶ Go for lean white meat or, better still, fish.

▶ Choose grilled fish, chicken or vegetables rather than fried dishes.

▶ Beware vegetarian options – they may look healthy but are often laden with cheese and cream.

▶ Don't be afraid to ask for a small portion.

▶ Fill your plate with vegetables rather than potatoes, rice or pasta.

▶ Stick to two starters or one main course.

▶ Don't even look at the dessert menu.

Jane Wisdom

Pub-food portions tend to be larger than those in restaurants. You may need to cut back your portion size by more than a third.

WHAT'S YOUR FAVOURITE RESTAURANT?

You can still enjoy a wide range of foods while keeping calories, fat and salt under control. Here's how:

Italian

If you avoid pasta and pizza, it's easy to make healthy choices.

Choose:

▶ Melon and Parma ham – a delicious low-calorie starter.

▶ Rocket salad – high in iron and very low in calories.

▶ Grilled fish, meat or vegetables.

▶ Tomato-based sauces, as they tend to be lower in calories.

Avoid:

▶ Pasta and risotto dishes but if you can't resist them, share your portion with a friend or ask for a starter size.

▶ Creamy sauces combined with meat-based dishes, such as lasagne, which are high in calories.

▶ Pizza and bruschetta, but if you can't resist them, stick to a couple of slices – and don't eat the crusts.

▶ Desserts with mascarpone – just say no.

French

Simply cooked French food is healthy and delicious, but try to avoid the more complicated dishes and creamy sauces.

Choose:

▶ Grilled fish.

▶ Salad and vegetables to fill up your plate.

▶ Grilled steak, as long as it's the size of your iPhone – a real treat and a great source of iron.

▶ Simple soups, but say no to bread.

Avoid:

▶ Frites and pommes dauphinoise.

▶ Creamy sauces – they are high in calories and saturated fat.

▶ Garlic bread – pretend you're a vampire.

▶ Moules marinières – it's impossible to enjoy them without dipping in bread or fries.

▶ Cheeses – both hard and soft cheeses are high in fat and calories.

▶ Dessert – need I say more!

Indian and Chinese

Indian and Chinese meals are often loaded with saturated fat and salt so should ideally be avoided. If you choose carefully, however, and monitor your portion control, they can be low in calories.

Choose:

▶ Baked dishes from the tandoor oven such as chicken tikka or shashlik.

▶ Plain boiled rice, but only a tennis-ball-sized portion.

▶ Stir-fried vegetables.

Avoid:

▶ All sauces, particularly the creamier ones such as korma.

▶ Coconut might sound healthy, but it is very high in calories.

▶ Naan breads, poppadoms, stuffed paratha and prawn crackers – all are high in calories.

▶ Onion bhajees, samosas and spring rolls are deep-fried and high in saturated fat.

▶ Fried dishes, such as sweet-and-sour pork.

STILL STRUGGLING?

Don't forget your visual reminders:

▶ Alerts on your mobile.

▶ Calorie-counting apps.

▶ Post-its on your computer.

DRINK WISELY

▶ Drink plenty of water throughout the meal.

▶ A slimline tonic with ice and a slice of lemon is a great pre-dinner drink.

▶ Go for a spritzer – it has only half the calories of two glasses of wine and lasts the same amount of time.

▶ Alternate every sip of wine with a few sips of water.

▶ Volunteer to be the driver.

■

Chapter Twelve

SKINNY RULE 8: MOVE MORE

THE BEAUTY OF the Jane Plan way of life is that it not only helps you lose weight by making dietary changes, but it also helps you make lifestyle changes to ensure you keep it off for good. Although it is important to cut back on your daily calories, it is also important to increase your physical activity. The reason? Eating provides calories, whereas activity burns them off, so the more you move the more calories you will burn.

Being active is not just about losing weight and shaping up, however, although that is one of the big bonuses. It also helps you to become more energetic as well as instilling an overall sense of well-being. There is another plus point too: muscle burns more calories than non-muscle tissue – even when you are sitting down. As you gain more muscle by being more active – provided you stick to the Skinny Rules – your body will become even more efficient at getting energy from food. Last but not least, exercise will help you become more body aware so that you won't want to stoke it up with unhealthy foods.

Jane Wisdom
Research shows that an active lifestyle is crucial for successful weight loss and even more critical for long-term weight maintenance.

The good news is that being more active doesn't necessarily mean scheduling strenuous workouts in the gym; you may be too busy, too tired or simply not confident enough to join. A combination of walking, resistance training and just being more active as you go about your daily life can be beneficial. The important thing is to get moving – every step you take counts, whether it's cleaning the house, climbing the stairs rather than taking the lift or getting off the bus one stop earlier.

Jane Wisdom
Note down how much activity you do each day in your food diary. Research suggests that people who keep track of their activity levels as well as what they eat are more successful in the weight-loss game than those who don't.

GET MOVING

Although very active people can burn up to 30 per cent of their calories through daily activities, for most of us, especially if we are sedentary, it can be as low as 15 per cent. Most office workers, for example, are sedentary – so this could be you! Don't kid yourself that just because you walk to the bus stop every day you aren't sedentary – if you sit at a desk for eight hours a day, you almost certainly are!

Simply being aware of this fact, and taking every opportunity to move, can make a dramatic difference to the amount of calories you burn.

At Jane Plan, we try to keep a 'keep moving' message in our minds at all times. It sounds silly, but it works. Write down the words 'move more' and 'ideas on how to do it' on Post-it notes and put them where you'll notice them when you're sitting still. At Jane Plan HQ we pop them on our computers and follow them whenever we can.

Here are some ideas we use that work:

▶ Tap your feet

▶ Swing your legs

▶ Drum your fingers

▶ Stand up and stretch

▶ Move your head from side to side

▶ Change position

▶ Wriggle around

▶ Pace up and down

▶ Stand up every time the phone rings

▶ Don't use an internal phone – get up and speak to someone

▶ Use the loo on another floor

▶ Clench and release your muscles

You'll be amazed at the opportunities you find to burn more calories if you remember to keep your eye out for them. *Keep* thinking, *keep* moving.

Now you've conquered moving in your seat, it's time to get moving in your everyday life too. Experts recommend that you walk about 10,000 steps a day. Here are some ideas to ease yourself gently into exercise:

► Take the stairs rather than the escalator or lift.

► Walk the children to school.

► Park at least a 10-minute walk from your front door.

► Walk around the house during the TV ad breaks.

► Rather than emailing the person at the next-door desk, get up and go and talk to them.

► Go for a walk around the block or in the local park during your lunch hour.

► Play football with the children, go dancing or bowling rather than watching TV or going to the cinema.

► Keep a pair of trainers or some comfy shoes in your bag by the front door – they will help you walk further, faster.

Jane Wisdom

As you start to move more, not only will you burn more calories but you will also start to feel more energised, self-confident and relaxed.

PEDOMETER POWER

A pedometer is an easy way to track your progress. Remember that it takes a deficit of 3,500 calories to burn a pound (450g) of fat, so if you aim to burn an extra 250 calories a day through walking that's an additional half-pound (225g) weight loss a week. Check the chart below to see how many calories you can expect to burn by taking a 15-minute walk; however, remember that exericise only acts an effective weight-loss tool when *combined with a calorie-controlled diet.* Eating the Jane Plan way and exercising regularly will help you on your weight-loss journey

Body weight	Calories burned on a 15-minute walk
140lb (10 stone)	74
160lb (11 stone 6lb)	85
180lb (12 stone 12lb)	94
200lb (14 stone 4lb)	106
220lb (15 stone 10lb)	117
240lb (17 stone 2lb)	128
260lb (18 stone 7lb)	138
280lb (20 stone)	149
300lb (21 stone 6lb)	160
320lb (22 stone 12lb)	170
340lb-plus (24 stone 4lb-plus)	181-plus

Jane Wisdom

Don't drive to the gym. Have a Boris moment and cycle. Adding these few minutes of exercise before you arrive means you can ditch the warm-up, saving you valuable time.

STEPPING UP YOUR ACTIVITY LEVELS

Once you've adopted a more active lifestyle, you might like to think about adding some more activities. The secret is to choose something you enjoy. That way it is less likely to become a chore and you are more likely to stick with it. The best exercise plan, however, should incorporate a combination of cardio, resistance training and stretching. Around 30 minutes of moderate-intensity exercise at least five days a week is what the experts recommend as a minimum for most people, but remember: the harder and longer you exercise the more calories you will burn.

Cardio This is any activity that burns calories and helps to strengthen your heart. Walking, running, dancing, swimming and cycling are all good choices.

Resistance Lifting light weights with high repetition will help to tone your body and increase bone density, reducing your risk of osteoporosis. Lifting heavy weights will help you build more muscle – and remember: muscles burn more energy than fat. For every pound of muscle you gain you will burn an extra 20–45 calories a day. A recent study showed that regular resistance training can boost basal metabolic rate by 15 per cent. The reason? Muscle is metabolically active and burns more calories than other body tissue even when you are not moving.

Sit-ups, press-ups and exercises using light weights are good ways to start resistance training. As you get more confident and stronger, you should start upping the weights to maintain progress.

Stretching after every workout helps prevent injury and keeps you flexible. It is also great for balancing the body and mind.

Jane Wisdom

People who reward themselves are more likely to stay active long-term. How about a massage or simply an hour of 'me time'?

THE HEALTH GAINS OF EXERCISE

Research shows that increasing your daily activity can help to:

► Lower blood pressure

► Reduce cholesterol

► Prevent osteoporosis by increasing bone density

► Reduce the risk of type-2 diabetes

► Reduce the risk of some cancers

► Improve blood sugar control

► Enhance mental well-being

CAN YOU EXERCISE OFF THAT TREAT?

In terms of exercise, this is what and how much you need to do to burn off the following foods:

Food	Activity
1 large lasagne (560 cals)	45-minute spinning class
Chocolate muffin (476 cals)	58 minutes climbing
Packet of crisps (184 cals)	35 minutes playing Frisbee

→

Food	Activity
Tuna and mayo sandwich (310 cals)	70-minute body-pump class
Bacon sandwich (430 cals)	58 minutes playing football
Ham, egg on toast (436 cals)	90 minutes playing netball
Granny Smith apple (62 cals)	15 minutes resistance training
Mars bar	50 minutes aquarobics
Glass of juice (160 calls)	20 minutes skipping
Large glass of wine	20 minutes Zumba

Jane Wisdom

Go shopping. A Debenhams' survey of 2,000 women found that on average women take 7,300 steps per shopping trip – close to the recommended 10,000 a day. On average you need to walk 20 steps to burn one calorie, so that's 365 calories burnt on a shopping trip with the girls.

Jane Wisdom

Whether you're off on a picnic, a walk or a day out, turn your park into your personal gym and involve the whole family in calorie-burning activities. A game of Frisbee, rounders, volleyball, tennis, hide-and-seek or a long bike ride are all great options. Just remember that an hour of activity can burn as many as 300 calories.

Part Three

■

INSIDE THE
JANE PLAN KITCHEN

Many diets are unsustainable, faddy and don't fit in with a busy life. We do things differently in the Jane Plan kitchen. Our way of cooking and eating is fad-free, nutritionally balanced, and is also practical and delicious.

In this section there are lots of recipe ideas, all portion and calorie controlled especially for you, plus sample menus and skinny snack suggestions to inspire and keep you on the right track. You'll also find at-a-glance calorie counter charts to help you stick within your daily limit so you succeed in reaching your weight-loss goal.

Chapter Thirteen

■

GET TO KNOW YOUR FOODS

THE BASIC PRINCIPLE of the Jane Plan way of eating is that you can eat anything you like. Nothing is banned – except, of course, the biscuit tin. All the major food groups – protein, fat and carbohydrates – are included in the correct balance.

There are a few essentials, however. The first is calorie and portion control, and the second is that you buy the best-quality food you can afford. Last but not least, I also recommend that you opt for a plant-strong diet with plenty of fresh vegetables and fruit. Don't worry, though, shopping the Jane Plan way won't necessarily add pounds to your weekly shopping bill because you will be buying smaller quantities than you currently do. Down to the specifics, I recommend:

1. You aim to eat around 1,000–1,200 calories a day depending on your BMR.

2. You eat three meals a day with two healthy snacks in between.

3. You practise a carb curfew (no carbs after 4.00pm) in the early stages of your diet.

WHAT TO EAT

As you start to follow the Jane Plan recipes, you will be including a variety of nutrient-rich foods from the main food groups to ensure your diet is as healthy and as balanced as possible, but first I am going to tell you a little more about the various food groups and the role they play in the Jane Plan kitchen.

Carbohydrates

Many weight-loss plans are based on restricting or cutting out carbs altogether. But carbs provide the same amount of calories per gram as protein and, as long as you go for the right type, they provide you with much-needed energy. The trouble is that many of us eat too many. Why? Because carbs are moreish and many popular foods are carb-based. As a result, the weight goes on, but this is due to eating excess calories rather than a high-carb diet.

You know how easy it is to sit down to a plate piled high with delicious pasta – probably far more than you really need – and before you've even noticed it you've finished the lot! And it doesn't stop at pasta – toast is just the same (one slice never seems to be enough).

Jane Wisdom
Carbs need to be treated with caution.

Making the right choice

When eating carbs, go for the types found in foods such as por-ridge oats, whole-wheat pasta, brown rice, pearl barley and wholegrain breakfast cereals. They're not lower in calories than the more refined types, but they do take longer to digest and have a low GI (glycaemic index). This is a way of rating foods according to how fast they can be digested and converted to glucose – your body's energy source. Foods with a high GI cause a rapid rise in blood sugar levels, whereas those with a lower rating result in a steadier more gradual rise, which means they help to keep your blood sugar levels stable and keep you feeling fuller for longer. The result? You eat less and increase your chances of successful weight loss. And these are the type of carbs we mostly use at Jane Plan. The secret is: think whole-grain and brown rather than white and refined.

Problems can arise if you eat too many high-GI carbs found in sugary sweet foods, such as biscuits or puddings. The reason? They have a high glycaemic index, which provides a quick surge of energy to the body, but this peak is short lived, and as soon it subsides the body usually starts to crave another high-glycaemic food for a repeat energy fix. This can trigger a cycle of energy peaks and troughs, which in turn can lead to overeating and weight gain.

Go on a carb curfew

An easy and effective way to curb your carb overload is to follow a carb curfew, especially in the early stages of your diet. The reason? It will naturally help you limit your calorie intake and steer you towards a plant-based diet as you replace carbo-hydrates with extra vegetables.

It's up to you what time you start your carb curfew – I like to start mine at 4.00pm. It stops me nibbling on carbs (confession time – I'm tempted by biscuits) when the children come home from school, or having a late-afternoon biscuit break with a cup of tea when I am working.

Whatever time you start, a carb curfew will help to stop you reaching for that bag of crisps after work or going for a mountain of pasta at dinner, and make you focus on new choices. Like everything on Jane Plan, see this as an opportunity to sample new things, rather than an exercise in cutting back.

Don't be put off by the idea of a carb curfew – you may enjoy it so much that you never eat carbs again in the evenings. If, however, you start to miss that plate of pasta or risotto for dinner, you can re-introduce them once you have reached your goal weight, but always with an eye on portion control. I explain all about portion control in Skinny Rule 3, page 76.

COUNT THEM OUT

The main food groups provide the body with calories, but in different amounts. Although you probably know that fats contain more calories than other food groups you may be surprised to learn that carbohydrates and protein contain the same amount of calories and that alcohol has almost as many calories as fat.

Here's how many calories are in 1g of each:

Carbohydrate: 4 calories

Protein: 4 calories

Fat: 9 calories

Alcohol: 7 calories

Protein

Protein is often touted as 'the dieter's friend'. The reason? It keeps you feeling fuller for longer and helps build muscle tissue (and remember, muscle burns more calories than any other tissue). And that's not all. Digesting protein uses up more calories than digesting other nutrients. These are all reasons they are included in just the right amount in the Jane Plan way of eating. But don't think that magically eating protein will make you lose weight, because it won't.

Remember: protein has the same amount of calories as carbohydrates (see box on the previous page).

Protein is usually associated with meat, chicken and fish, but pulses, seeds and soya products, such as tofu, are all rich sources too and feature high in the Jane Plan way of eating.

The following are all good sources of protein:

White meat Go for organic or free-range chicken wherever possible. The meat from battery-bred chickens is usually pumped with water and, if press reports are anything to go by, a lot of other nasties too. The meat can also be higher in fat as a result of the chickens' sedentary lifestyle. Whichever type you choose, remove the skin and eat the white rather than the darker meat, because this is lower in fat.

Red meat Red meat is an excellent source of protein and iron. When you do eat it always go for the best quality you can afford and look for 'grass-fed and pasture-raised' on labels, because these meats have higher levels of healthy omega-3 fats (see page 125). Cut off any visible fat and pour away fatty juices after cooking. Grill rather than fry. And try venison – it's just as delicious as beef and is a healthy lean meat.

Jane Wisdom

If you are a red-meat lover, try to stick to no more than 70g a day in accordance with the Food Standards Agency guidelines and open up your repertoire to other sources of protein such as fish, eggs and pulses.

Fish At Jane Plan we love fish – it's full of protein, plus a wide variety of vitamins and minerals and the all-important omega-3 fats, which studies show help reduce inflammation in the body and lower the risk of heart disease, diabetes and many other conditions. Although oily fish, such as tuna and salmon, is higher in fat, and therefore calories, than other fish, it still features in the Jane Plan way of eating on account of its huge health benefits, and it is an important part of any healthy diet.

Eggs Not just for breakfast, eggs are a complete meal in themselves. A rich source of protein, they really do keep you feeling full for longer. Full of vitamins, including vitamin A and many B vitamins such as folic acid, very few foods share the same diverse nutrient make-up. Best of all, an egg is already portion controlled for you – you don't have to do a thing!

Peas, beans, lentils These are all excellent sources of fibre and protein as well as being low in fat. They are also rich in folic acid, copper, iron and magnesium – nutrients that many of us are missing out on in our diets. Don't be afraid to eat the tinned versions. They are über-convenient, especially after a long, hard day.

Nuts They may be full of fibre and protein, but nuts can be high in fat and calories as well. What's more, nuts are moreish, and it can be hard to stick to just a handful. When watching your calories, it is best to count them out one by one rather than just grabbing a handful! My Skinny Snacks list, page 146, tells you how many nuts to eat as a snack.

Seeds High in omega-3 fats, these make a great addition to salads, but remember that even a handful counts towards your total calorie count.

Eat veg first, then fruit

You will notice that vegetables always come before fruit on Jane Plan. That's because, although fruits are packed with goodness, some are high in sugar (fructose) and calories. Vegetables, on the other hand, contain loads of fibre and generally far less sugar.

What's more, a large portion of vegetables, especially the green kind, can clock up just 30 cals. Now you can understand why I like to think veg, then fruit. The calorie chart on page 269 will tell you the most weight-friendly ones to choose.

PUT A RAINBOW ON YOUR PLATE

The pigmented chemicals, also known as phytonutrients, which give fruit and vegetables their colour, have a host of health benefits ranging from boosting immunity to protecting against some forms of cancer. The best way to ensure you get the most from them is to pile your plate high with many different-coloured varieties.

PUT A RAINBOW ON YOUR PLATE

Colour	Choose	Why?
Red	Beetroot, red onion, red pepper, red-skinned potatoes, tomatoes, cherries, cranberries, pomegranate, red and pink grapefruit, red grapes, watermelon	For lycopene, which is a powerful carotenoid found in red, orange and yellow veg. Carotenoids are turned into the antioxidant vitamin A in the body, one of the 'big three' ACE vitamins, which help guard against free-radical damage
Orange	Carrots, orange pepper, sweet potatoes, butternut squash, apricots, cantaloupe melon, mango, papaya	Carotenoids are the key ingredients in orange fruit and veg. Other important ingredients include bioflavonoids, a large group of chemical compounds, which, according to research, decrease inflammation and work in various ways to stop or slow the development of cancer, heart disease and neurodegenerative diseases
Yellow	Yellow pepper, sweetcorn, yellow pumpkin, grapefruit, lemon, peach, pineapple	For carotenoids (see above). Yellow fruit and veg are also good sources of two compounds, lutein and zeaxanthin, which are major pigments in the eye. Studies show that consuming higher amounts of lutein and zeaxanthin in the diet lowers the risk of developing age-related macular degeneration (AMD)

→

Colour	Choose	Why?
Green	Artichoke, asparagus, broccoli, Brussels sprouts, cabbage, celery, green beans, green pepper, curly kale, pak choi and other leafy greens, avocado, apple, grapes, honeydew melon, kiwi fruit, lime	Chlorophyll, the chemical responsible for giving plants their green colour, may help to quell inflammation, prevent cell mutation and strengthen immunity. Vegetables such as broccoli, Brussels sprouts, cabbage, kale and pak choi are also sources of indole-3 carbinols, compounds that may help protect against some types of cancer
Blue, indigo and violet	Aubergine, cabbage, purple-fleshed potatoes, bilberries, blackberries, blueberries, Victoria plums, purple and black grapes	All are rich sources of anthocyanins, which may help preserve memory and cognitive function as we age

I'm not suggesting that your diet should be 100 per cent vegetables, but making a few simple changes such as introducing meat-free Mondays is a great way to make positive changes to your diet. It's an opportunity to do something different, cook and eat different foods and experience new flavours. Studies also suggest that a plant-strong diet might help reduce the risk of conditions such as heart disease and diabetes. If you are wondering how to ensure you have enough protein on your meat-free Mondays include nuts, pulses (beans, chickpeas and lentils) and quinoa too.

Jane Wisdom

Fresh fruit is best. You should always eat more fresh than dried fruit. Dried fruit is higher in calories by volume. A cup of raisins (which are dried grapes), for example, contains more calories than a cup of grapes, because there are more of them per cup.

Fats

Not all fats are equal, but the right fats are an essential part of the Jane Plan way of eating. Just as with protein and carbs, however, the appropriate fats should be eaten strictly in the right amounts.

'Bad' saturated fats found in red meat and dairy may increase the risk of heart disease and bowel cancer, and trans-fats and hydrogenated fats found in shop-bought biscuits, pastries and margarine and other manufactured foods raise cholesterol levels and have been linked to heart disease and cancer risk.

According to a study published in the *New England Medical Journal*, calorie for calorie, trans-fats increase the risk of heart disease more than any other major nutrient, even at a low intake. Research also suggests that eating trans-fats may result in a higher risk of other health problems, including Alzheimer's disease, diabetes, fat around the middle and infertility. The good news is that recently the quantity of trans-fats has been reduced in processed foods, but the bad news is that if there is less than 0.5 per cent, manufacturers don't need to state this on the label, so small amounts can still remain but not be noted. My advice is that it's best to leave these types of food off the shopping list for good.

On the other hand 'good' unsaturated fats (the type we mostly use at Jane Plan), found in nuts, seeds and their oils as well as oily fish and olive oil are a rich source of essential fatty acids, which have a host of health benefits.

The great dairy debate

Dairy has an important part to play in any healthy diet, but if you are dairy intolerant, don't worry. There are lots of dairy substitutes around, such as rice milk, soya milk, almond milk and oat milk. Always check the labels before buying, though, as they often contain sweeteners. At Jane Plan we recommend:

▶ Half-fat crème fraîche or fromage frais.

▶ No-fat, or low-fat, Greek yogurt (it's deliciously thick and creamy and will help you feel more satisfied – it's also unsweetened).

▶ Lower calorie cheeses, such as goat's cheese.

▶ Skimmed or 1 per cent milk.

Anti-dairy? Go for soya, rice or oat milk. But be a conscious calorie counter – not all non-dairy milks are low in calories. Soya milks, for example, are often sweetened. Look for unsweetened varieties.

Jane Wisdom

If you are worried about your calcium levels and don't like dairy, broccoli, kale and other green, leafy vegetables are great sources of calcium.

Jane Wisdom
If you're a fruit lover, choose berries – they have fewer calories, less sugar and won't affect your blood sugar levels as much as some other fruits, such as bananas. I am not anti bananas but they should be enjoyed in moderation.

Seasoning

Many of us eat too much salt, which can raise blood pressure and with it the risk of associated health problems. That's why as soon as you start to eat the Jane Plan way you will be using very little salt in your cooking, and some of the recipes are salt-free. Instead, you will be using herbs and spices to enhance flavour.

If you are used to eating highly seasoned food, add a tiny sprinkle of salt and aim to reduce the amount you add every day. You will soon get used to the taste of less seasoned and healthier food. Six grams a day is the maximum recommended intake of salt, which is about one teaspoon.

When it comes to pepper, however, you can be generous. Freshly ground pepper is a wonderful complement to food – try black, white and green peppercorns.

Jane Wisdom
Use chilli to spice up your food – it's thought to help weight loss, as it acts as an appetite suppressant.

Water

I recommend you have approximately 1.5 litres of water a day. Thirst can be mistaken for hunger, so good hydration can help to curb hunger. In turn, this means that you are less likely to snack and, if you drink a large glass of water before meal times, you'll feel fuller. Treat water as your new best friend – never leave home without your bottle.

To make plain tap water more appetising simply fill a jug and add frozen lemon and lime slices, fresh mint leaves or a handful of colourful berries.

Tea and coffee

You can drink tea and filter coffee with a splash of skimmed milk, but you may want to reduce the amount, as caffeine alters blood sugar levels. If you usually add sugar, try going without, or use a sweetener. Despite the scare stories of how sweeteners might actually trigger weight gain and even cancer, unless you use sweeteners in huge quantities they are unlikely to affect your weight or your health. You can have unlimited herbal teas. Enjoy exploring the different flavours available. Camomile is calming, valerian will help you sleep, peppermint aids digestion while lemon and ginger will boost your get up and go.

Low calorie/diet drinks

You can have low-calorie fizzy drinks and sugar-free squash, but not too many – try fizzy mineral water instead. Research suggests that people who do opt for low-cal fizzy drinks do not necessarily consume fewer calories overall.

Juices

It's best to avoid fruit juices altogether – they are high in sugar and calories.

We don't juice or make smoothies at Jane Plan, and the reasons are twofold:

1. As soon as you peel a piece of fruit or vegetable you remove the goodness, because much of it is found in the skin.

2. How often do you eat three apples at a time? Juicing tends to make you eat more fruit than you normally would.

Eat one piece of fruit and have a glass of water instead of juicing.

Alcohol

Alcohol is high in calories and after a couple of drinks you may lose your 'diet resolve'. If you really can't go without a glass of wine, try to have a detox on your first Jane Plan week and give it up completely – a week's not that long! Then re-introduce a small glass at the weekends only. See Skinny Rule 6 on page 99.

Jane Wisdom

Cutting back on alcohol isn't just good for your waistline, it's good for your health too.

Chapter Fourteen

.

ESSENTIALLY YOURS

A WELL-STOCKED store cupboard, fridge and freezer make eating and cooking the Jane Plan way a whole lot easier. Here are some suggestions for what to keep in your Jane Plan kitchen to make your meals fresh, fun and interesting. A bit of wasabi or horseradish sauce, for example, can really perk up a simple fish lunch.

IN THE STORE CUPBOARD

Sea salt (preferably Maldon)

Black peppercorns

Dijon mustard

English mustard

Wholegrain mustard

Olive oil

Groundnut oil

Honey

Balsamic vinegar

White wine vinegar

Soy sauce

Fish sauce

Wasabi

Dried chilli flakes

Mirin

Mixed herbs and spices

Harissa

Tahini paste

Tamarind paste

Capers

Olives

Tomato puree

Sun-dried tomatoes

Anchovies

Curry powder

Thai curry paste

Tabasco

Bottles of water

Sugar-free muesli

Pure porridge oats

Almonds

Pistachio nuts

Hazelnuts

Walnuts

Dried goji berries

Pumpkin seeds

Pine nuts

Sunflower seeds

Herbal teas

Chicken, beef, lamb, fish and
vegetable stock cubes

Canned chickpeas, lentils, kidney
beans, aduki beans and butter
beans

Canned tomatoes

Dried Puy lentils

Aduki beans

Vermouth

Dried porcini (ceps)

Horseradish

Gherkins

Quinoa

Optional extras:

Rice noodles

Pasta

Basmati rice

Couscous

Rye crackers

Crispbreads

Oatcakes

Rice cakes

Miso soup

IN THE FRIDGE

Low-fat natural Greek yoghurt

Low-fat crème fraîche

Low-fat fromage frais

Feta cheese/halloumi/ricotta
cheese/mozzarella

Semi-skimmed or skimmed milk

Parma ham

Fresh berries in season:
blueberries, raspberries,
strawberries

Parmesan

Hummus, tzatzki, cottage cheese

Rocket

Watercress

Salad leaves

Cucumber

Tomatoes

Radishes

Spring onions

Chicory

Celery

Asparagus

Pak choi

Fennel

Peppers

Eggs

Smoked salmon

Prawns

Mini chicken fillets

Fresh herbs – basil, coriander, parsley, dill, chives, tarragon, mint

Fresh root ginger

Lemongrass

Fresh chilli

IN THE FREEZER

Berries

Broad beans

Peas

Sorbet

Soups

Chicken breasts/mini fillets/thighs

Bag of mixed seafood

Minced beef

Beef for braising

Lamb for braising

Salmon steaks, smoked mackerel fillets, cod fillets, plaice fillets

Prawns

Kaffir lime leaves

IN THE VEGETABLE BASKET

Broccoli

Beans

Mangetouts

Spinach

Carrots

Artichokes

Courgettes

Cauliflower

Aubergine

Squash

Potatoes

Sweet potato

Onions   Red onions
Banana shallots   Mushrooms
Garlic   Beetroot

IN THE FRUIT BOWL

Lemons   Kiwi fruit
Limes   Passion fruit
Oranges   Satsumas
Apples   Clementines
Pears   Figs
Peaches   Tropical fruits: mango/
Nectarines   pineapple (for a
Plums   weekend treat only)

Jane Wisdom

Check your store cupboard, fridge, freezer and fruit bowl at regular intervals throughout the week and replenish as necessary. This ensures you always have healthy ingredients to hand, which reduces the risk of naughty nibbling.

Chapter Fifteen

■

YOUR JANE PLAN
WEEKLY MENU PLANNER

S IMPLE GOOD FOOD that is easy to prepare is integral to the Jane Plan way of eating, so here's a week of sample menus to get you started. The menus are between 1,000 and 1,200 calories, but they don't include extra milk for teas and coffees. They are also based on very exact measurements, so if you add an extra potato or even a splash of salad dressing, the calorie counts will go up.

Following a 1,000–1,200 calorie-a-day plan works well and delivers a sustainable weight loss without leaving you feeling hungry or deprived. But remember: if you want to be 100 per cent accurate about how many calories you should be eating each day in order to meet your weight-loss goals, you'll need to revisit the BMR details on page 47–48 and get your calculator out.

MONDAY

BREAKFAST
Very Berry Porridge (page 159)
Total: 246 calories

MID MORNING
1 medium apple
Total: 77 calories

LUNCH
Spinach and Rocket Soup: 286 calories (page 167)
A small (55g) pot of fromage frais: 47 calories
(optional)

Total: 333 calories

MID AFTERNOON
9 almonds
Total: 88 calories

DINNER
Chilli Tuna Steak (page 213) with watercress
and roasted vine tomatoes
Total: 421 calories

Daily calories: 1,173

TUESDAY

BREAKFAST
Apple, Cinnamon and Walnut Whip with yoghurt
(page 164)
Total: 181 calories

MID MORNING
1 rye cracker with 30g low-fat soft cheese
Total: 105 calories

LUNCH
Quinoa, Crudités and Parmesan Salad (page 179)
Total: 349 calories

MID AFTERNOON
1 nectarine
Total: 54 calories

DINNER
Lemony Lamb with Rosemary, Mint and Broad Beans:
300 calories (page 230)
Mixed salad: 30 calories
1 tbsp olive oil and balsamic vinegar dressing: 67 calories
100g new potatoes: 75 calories (optional)
Total: 472 calories (with potatoes)
Total: 397 calories (without potatoes)

Daily calories: 1,161 (with potatoes) or
1,086 (without potatoes)

WEDNESDAY

BREAKFAST
Nutritious Nut Porridge (page 161)
Total: 304 calories

MID MORNING
1 medium banana
Total: 142 calories

LUNCH
Red Lentil, Chickpea and Chilli Soup (page 170)
Total: 343 calories

MID AFTERNOON
1 celery stick with 1 tbsp cottage cheese
Total: 21 calories

DINNER
The Mediterranean One: 268 calories
(page 224)
Mixed salad of endive, radicchio, green leaves and
herbs: 30 calories
1 tbsp olive oil and balsamic vinegar dressing:
67 calories
Total: 365 calories

Daily calories: 1,175

THURSDAY

BREAKFAST
Scrambled Eggs with Parma Ham, made with 2 eggs
(page 151)
Total: 221 calories

MID MORNING
2 clementines or 1 orange
Total: 70 calories (clementines)
Total: 62 calories (orange)

LUNCH
Warm Halloumi Salad with Chilli Dressing (page 191)
Total: 383 calories

MID AFTERNOON
1 low-fat strawberry yoghurt
Total: 79 calories

DINNER
Warm Roasted Vegetable Salad: 217 calories (page 206)
½ grilled chicken breast: 96 calories
1 tsp pesto: 50 calories
Total: 363 calories

Daily calories: 1,116 with clementines or
1,108 with orange

FRIDAY

BREAKFAST
Beautiful Banana Porridge (page 160)
Total: 334 calories

MID MORNING
¼ pot of olives (average deli pot weighs 150g)
Total: 85 calories

LUNCH
Thai Chicken and Courgette Soup (page 189)
Total: 180 calories
or
Fig, Fennel and Parma Ham Salad (page 180)
Total: 154 calories

MID AFTERNOON
1 large carrot
Total: 28 calories

DINNER
Seafood Risotto (page 246)
Total: 601 calories

Daily calories: 1,228 (with Thai Chicken
and Courgette Soup)
or
1,202 (with Fig, Fennel and Parma Ham Salad)

SATURDAY

BREAKFAST
Baked Eggs with Spinach (page 154)
Total: 316 calories

MID MORNING
3 dried apricots
Total: 38 calories

LUNCH
Moroccan Chickpea Soup with Harissa (page 184)
Total: 159 calories

MID AFTERNOON
1 Babybel cheese
Total: 70 calories

DINNER
Sea Bream with Mexican Salsa (page 244)
Total: 582 calories

Daily calories: 1,165

SUNDAY

BREAKFAST
A Full English (page 156)
Total: 152 calories

MID MORNING
2 handfuls of blueberries
Total: 45 calories

LUNCH
Oriental Pork with Sweet Potato and Butternut
Squash: 562 calories (page 256)
Steamed spinach: 41 calories
Total: 603 calories

MID AFTERNOON
1 handful of grapes
Total: 51 calories

DINNER
Warm Asparagus Niçoise (page 200)
Total: 254 calories

Daily calories: 1,105

Chapter Sixteen

—

SKINNY SNACKS, MINI MOUTHFULS AND HARMLESS HANDFULS

S NACKING THE Jane Plan way doesn't mean you'll be grazing throughout the day, or absent-mindedly nibbling at your desk, but it does mean you'll be eating two well-chosen snacks each day, ideally one mid morning and one mid afternoon. As I know only too well, the problem with snacking is that it's very hard not to snack 'too much', so here are some super-convenient, portion- and calorie-controlled snacks for you to choose from.

SKINNY SNACKS

- ► 1 medium apple: 77 calories
- ► 1 rye cracker with 30g low-fat soft cheese: 105 calories
- ► 1 rounded tbsp tzatziki, plus a handful of crudités: 60 calories
- ► 1 low-fat strawberry yoghurt (110g pot): 79 calories

- ► 1 oatcake spread with a cheese triangle: 82 calories
- ► 1 medium banana: 142 calories
- ► ¼ deli pot of olives: 85 calories
- ► 1 orange: 62 calories
- ► 1 shop-bought mini pack of mango cubes: 46 calories
- ► 1 slice of cantaloupe melon: 34 calories
- ► 1 shop-bought apple and grape pack: 45 calories
- ► 2 clementines: 70 calories
- ► 1 large carrot: 28 calories
- ► 2 slices of Parma ham wrapped around a large celery stick: 43 calories
- ► 1 oatcake with Marmite: 37 calories
- ► 1 miso soup: 30 calories
- ► 1 nectarine: 54 calories
- ► 1 medium hard-boiled egg: 84 calories
- ► 1 stick of celery with 1 tbsp cottage cheese: 21 calories
- ► 2 rice cakes with 1 tbsp hummus: 97 calories

MINI MOUTHFULS

- ► 9 almonds: 88 calories
- ► 2 Brazil nuts: 82 calories
- ► 3 dried apricots: 38 calories
- ► 4 dates: 120 calories
- ► 2 walnuts: 91 calories

- ▶ 1 Babybel cheese: 70 calories
- ▶ 1 California sushi roll: 33 calories
- ▶ 1 mini box of raisins (Sunmaid's is 14g): 43 calories
- ▶ 1 square of Green & Black's dark chocolate: 22 calories
- ▶ 1 cheese triangle: 42 calories

HARMLESS HANDFULS

A handful is 80g of:

- ▶ Strawberries, plus 2 tbsp fat-free yoghurt: 83 calories
- ▶ Blackberries: 21 calories
- ▶ Cherries: 41 calories
- ▶ Crudités (carrot, pepper, cucumber): 27 calories
- ▶ Red grapes: 51 calories
- ▶ Cherry tomatoes: 14 calories
- ▶ Asparagus and a squeeze of lemon: 16 calories
- ▶ Raspberries: 22 calories
- ▶ Blueberries: 45 calories

A handful is 25g of:

- ▶ Mixed seeds: 150 calories

Jane Wisdom
Remember the phrase 'more than a handful's a waste'? It couldn't be truer than when it comes to snacking.

Chapter Seventeen

■

THE RECIPES

AS A BUSY WORKING woman and a mum of three, ease and convenience are my mantras when it comes to providing nourishing meals. The recipes that follow are simple dishes using everyday foods that I, my friends and my family, love to cook and eat. They are not necessarily 'diet' recipes, as I don't believe in diet food, just good food that is deliciously healthy and nutritionally balanced, as well as being calorie and portion controlled.

Eating is all about enjoyment, so don't be surprised to see small amounts of ingredients that you might not expect to find, such as butter, maple syrup and alcohol. As long as you factor them into your daily calorie allowance they won't damage your diet. Jane Plan eating is all about balancing calories – so provided you don't exceed your daily calorie limit, you can pick and choose whatever you like. It's as simple as that.

The recipes that follow will show you just how easy it is to eat delicious, healthy food and still lose weight. Enjoy.

BREAKFASTS

You often hear that breakfast is the most important meal of the day. Why? Because it kick-starts your metabolism, helps balance blood sugar levels and ensures you don't lose concentration halfway through the morning. Research also suggests that breakfast skippers are more likely to put on weight. That's because if you're hungry mid morning you risk making the wrong choices – cappuccino and a muffin are my downfall. If this sounds familiar, save yourself some calories and enjoy a balanced breakfast to help you start the day the right way.

I have divided my breakfast recipes into two sections: breakfasts for long, lazy mornings, when you have time to relax and really enjoy the first meal of the day, and breakfasts on the go, for those days when you are in such a rush you can easily forget to eat!

Breakfasts for long, lazy mornings

Eggs are a big part of the Jane Plan diet and make the perfect slimline breakfast, because they are already portion controlled as well as containing healthy fats, protein and lots of vitamins and minerals. The Jane Plan way of eating is also about buying the best-quality food you can afford, and there's no point in skimping on eggs. For a few pence extra you can buy free-range eggs: they are better for you, better for the chickens and they taste better too. All the following recipes can also be used for light lunches or simple suppers.

Scrambled Eggs and Parma Ham

SERVES 2   **CALS: 221** with 2 eggs; **145** with 1 egg

This is a great take on traditional bacon and eggs.

> 4 medium free-range eggs
> 1 tbsp skimmed milk
> a drop of olive oil
> 4 slices of Parma ham
> sea salt and freshly ground black pepper
> chopped fresh parsley leaves, to serve

Put the eggs into a bowl and whisk vigorously with the milk. Add a pinch of sea salt and a generous grind of pepper.

Add a drop of olive oil to a pan to lightly coat the base to prevent the eggs from sticking. Add the eggs and continue stirring as they gently cook.

Lay 2 slices of Parma ham on each plate and spoon the lightly scrambled eggs on top. Sprinkle with parsley and enjoy.

••

Jane Tip ≫ *This recipe also works well with smoked salmon and a squeeze of lemon, instead of the Parma ham.*

••

Soft Boiled Egg with Broccoli Soldiers

SERVES **2**   CALS: **104** with 1 egg; **180** with 2 eggs

Simple, delicious and low in calories, boiled eggs are the ideal family breakfast. You can feel secure, knowing exactly how many calories you are eating (with a boiled egg all the portion control is done for you) while hungry partners and children can enjoy them with traditional toasted soldiers.

> 1 handful of purple sprouting broccoli
> 1 or 2 medium free-range eggs
> sea salt and freshly ground black pepper

Trim the woody ends and tough leaves off the broccoli with a knife. Divide into small individual florets, each with a small stem – these are your soldiers. Put the broccoli soldiers into boiling water to cook, or steam, for 3–6 minutes until tender.

Put the eggs in a pan of cold water. Bring to the boil and simmer for 3–4 minutes. I like to put my egg in an eggcup and dip my broccoli soldiers into the yolk, but sometimes the broccoli spears are too thick for this. If that's the case, peel the egg, put it onto a plate and cut it in half, so that the lovely yolk spills gently out. Put the broccoli soldiers next to the egg and sprinkle with salt and pepper. Relax and enjoy dipping into your egg. Delicious!

···

Jane Tip » *You can use this recipe all year round using different seasonal vegetables. Broccoli spears are wonderful from February to April; come spring, you can change to asparagus! French beans and mangetouts also make great soldiers. If you like dipping the soldiers you'll find the asparagus and French beans work especially well.*

···

Poached Eggs with Smoked Salmon

SERVES **2**   CALS: **218** per serving, or **166** if you use half the amount of salmon

It's such a luxury having smoked salmon for breakfast, so why not spoil yourself occasionally?

   2 medium free-range eggs
   200g smoked salmon
   ¼ lemon, cut into two wedges
   freshly ground black pepper

Pour about 2.5cm boiling water into a small frying pan or saucepan. Return to the boil, reduce the heat to medium-high, then carefully crack the eggs into the pan, keeping them well apart. Cook for 3–5 minutes until done to your liking. (Alternatively, use an egg poacher according to the manufacturer's instructions.)

   Put the smoked salmon onto two serving plates and put your poached egg on top, then sprinkle with black pepper. Serve with the lemon.

· ·

Jane Tip » *I use a substantial amount of smoked salmon here, but if you want to cut the calories, use half the amount.*

· ·

Baked Eggs with Spinach

SERVES 2 CALS: 316 per serving

I love to serve this when I have friends over for brunch. It takes a little more time than the other breakfasts but is perfect for a long, lazy breakfast – café style! Spinach is brimming with iron, folate and a host of other vitamins and minerals.

  1 tbsp olive oil
  3 small onions, finely chopped
  500g fresh spinach
  4 tbsp semi-skimmed milk
  freshly grated nutmeg, to taste
  4 medium free-range eggs
  2 tbsp Parmesan cheese, finely grated
  freshly ground black pepper

Preheat the oven to 200°C/Gas 6. Heat the oil in a frying pan over a medium heat, add the onions and gently fry for 5–8 minutes until soft. Add the spinach, then cover and cook for 2–3 minutes or until wilted. Remove the lid and continue to cook until the liquid has evaporated.

Add the milk to the spinach and season with nutmeg and pepper. Spread the spinach mixture over the base of a shallow gratin dish and make four wells in the spinach with the back of a spoon.

Crack an egg into each well and sprinkle the cheese over the top. Bake for 12–15 minutes, or until the eggs are set. If you're not counting calories, serve with toasted granary bread.

Smoked Salmon Omelette

SERVES 2 CALS: 210 with 2 eggs per serving;
134 with 1 egg per serving

An omelette makes a filling breakfast and is perfect at the week-end, when you have more time on your hands. Use two eggs if you are looking for a substantial start to your day or one if you are holding back calories for lunch or dinner.

  4 medium free-range eggs
  50g frozen peas
  60g smoked salmon, chopped
  2 tsp fresh chopped tarragon leaves
  a little olive oil
  sea salt and freshly ground black pepper

Beat the eggs in a bowl. Add the peas, smoked salmon and tarragon, then season to taste. Pour the mixture into a lightly oiled shallow frying pan over a medium heat and cook until set around the edges. Lift the edges to allow the mixture to run underneath, then continue to cook until light and fluffy. Serve.

A Full English – The Jane Plan Way

SERVES **2** CALS: **152** per serving

The great thing about this breakfast is that you can enjoy a full English that's portion and calorie controlled while adding all sorts of extras for the rest of the family – and anyone else around who is not watching their weight. And it includes a rasher or two of bacon.

 2 large Portobello mushrooms
 a little olive oil
 2 large beef tomatoes
 2 thin rashers of back bacon with fat removed
 2 medium free-range eggs
 2 handfuls of watercress
 sea salt and freshly ground black pepper

Lightly brush the mushrooms with olive oil and add a touch of salt and pepper. Cut the tomatoes in half, season and put, skin-side down, under a hot grill, together with the mushrooms and bacon rashers.

Meanwhile, pour about 2.5cm boiling water into a small frying pan or saucepan. Return to the boil, reduce the heat to medium-high, crack the eggs open then carefully tip them into the pan, keeping them well apart. Cook for 3–5 minutes until done to your liking. (Alternatively, use an egg poacher according to the manufacturer's instructions.)

Put a handful of watercress on each plate, add the egg, mushroom, tomato and bacon rasher on top and season.

Jane Tip » *Add sausages, toast and other breakfast fare for your family, while you join in the fun with your skinny breakfast.*

Asparagus, Poached Eggs and Parmesan

SERVES **4** CALS: **313** per serving

This is a lovely way to start the day, and including Parmesan makes this brunch-style breakfast quite indulgent. But at 313 calories, it's a good idea to go for a lighter lunch to balance things out.

600g asparagus
8 medium free-range eggs
120g Parmesan cheese, shaved
sea salt and freshly ground black pepper

Snap off any woody ends from the asparagus stalks at the point where they break easily and discard. Bring a pan of water to the boil, add the asparagus, return it to the boil, then reduce the heat and simmer for 5 minutes or until tender.

Pour about 2.5cm boiling water into a small saucepan. Return to the boil, reduce the heat to medium-high, crack the eggs open then carefully tip them into the pan, keeping them well apart. Cook for 3–5 minutes until done to your liking. (Alternatively, use an egg poacher according to the manufacturer's instructions.)

Drain the asparagus in a colander and divide among four warmed plates. Top each plate with 2 eggs and scatter with the cheese. Season and serve.

Jane Tip » *This is lovely with roasted vine-ripened tomatoes. Put them in the oven at 200°C/Gas 6 before you start preparing the rest of the breakfast. No need to add oil! They should be ready at the same time as everything else. Non-dieters can enjoy the breakfast with rye bread.*

Grab-and-run breakfasts – for manic mornings

Most of us don't have time to think in the mornings, let alone cook. It's usually a case of opening the cupboard door, grabbing the first cereal you see and pouring it into a bowl while you boil the kettle, dry your hair and shout at the children. And if you haven't got children, you'll be checking your iPhone for the time of your first meeting. Whatever your lifestyle, weekday mornings can be manic, so I have put together some very simple grab-and-run breakfasts, which are quick and easy to make.

If you haven't time to make any of these recipes then make sure you buy a high-quality muesli, preferably sugar-free. Alara make delicious ones – they are mainly organic, often wheat-free and invariably sugar-free too. If you can't find Alara muesli, then get label savvy and read the nutritional information on other brands before buying. Alternatively, you can't go wrong with good old porridge oats.

Whether you choose muesli or porridge, make sure you pour no more than 40g – or about one 57 × 25mm ramekin – into your cereal bowl. Alternatively, grabbing a pot of yoghurt and an apple is an equally good and convenient breakfast.

Oat couture – five fun ways to cook porridge

The great thing about porridge is that it keeps you feeling full. But don't just have it in the winter – mix it with summer fruits, nuts and even dried fruits, and enjoy it all year round.

Here are five of my favourite ways to make porridge, but feel free to experiment and add your own fruits. As long as you stick to the portions given, you can't go far wrong on the calorie front. If you want to keep it simple, you don't need to add anything – porridge is perfect on its own. I prefer to cook my porridge in the microwave, because it only takes a few minutes.

1. Very Berry Porridge

SERVES 1 CALS: 246

> 40g porridge oats
> 200ml skimmed milk
> 1 tsp honey
> 80g mixed berries, such as raspberries, strawberries,
>   blueberries, blackberries

Put the porridge oats in a bowl. Cover with 180ml milk. Put in the microwave and cook for 1 minute. Stir, then cook for another 1 minute or until creamy, but keep checking – it sometimes needs less time, depending on the quality of your porridge oats and the strength of your microwave. (Alternatively, cook in the traditional way in a pan on the hob. Bring the mixture gently to the boil, then simmer for 5–10 minutes.) Once cooked, add a little more milk, stir in the honey and scatter over the berries before serving.

Jane Wisdom

Still wondering why porridge is so very good for you? It contains a considerable amount of fibre (soluble and insoluble), which is good for digestion. And as well as being an excellent low-GI food it contains beta glucans, which studies show may help reduce cholesterol levels.

If you are out and about don't worry. It is now much easier to buy porridge on the go.

2. Magnificent Mango Porridge

SERVES 1 **CALS: 271**

40g porridge oats
200ml skimmed milk
½ mango, cubed

Put the porridge oats in a bowl. Cover with 180ml milk. Put in the microwave and cook for 1 minute. Stir, then cook for another 1 minute or until creamy, but keep checking – it sometimes needs less time, depending on the quality of your porridge oats and the strength of your microwave. (Alternatively, cook in the traditional way in a pan on the hob. Bring the mixture gently to the boil, then simmer for 5–10 minutes.) Once cooked, add a little more milk and gently stir the mango into your porridge, then serve.

3. Beautiful Banana Porridge

SERVES 1 **CALS: 334**

40g porridge oats
200ml skimmed milk
1 banana, sliced

Put the porridge oats in a bowl. Cover with 180ml milk. Put in the microwave and cook for 1 minute. Stir, then cook for another 1 minute or until creamy, but keep checking – it sometimes needs less time, depending on the quality of your porridge oats and the strength of your microwave. (Alternatively, cook in the traditional way in a pan on the hob. Bring the mixture gently to the boil, then simmer for 5–10 minutes.) Once cooked, add a little more milk and put the banana slices on top. This makes a power-packed start to your day – great if you're working-out first thing.

4. Nutritious Nut Porridge

SERVES **1**   CALS: **304**

40g porridge oats
200ml skimmed milk
1 tsp honey
8 almonds, roughly chopped

Put the porridge oats in a bowl. Cover with 180ml milk. Put in the microwave and cook for 1 minute. Stir, then cook for another 1 minute or until creamy, but keep checking – it sometimes needs less time, depending on the quality of your porridge oats and the strength of your microwave. (Alternatively, cook in the traditional way in a pan on the hob. Bring the mixture gently to the boil, then simmer for 5–10 minutes.) Once cooked, add a little more milk and stir in the honey. Scatter the almonds on top for a great protein boost.

5. Gorgeous Goji Porridge

SERVES 1 **CALS: 266**

A so-called super food, goji berries are thought to have all sorts of health benefits, but the evidence is scanty. I use them with porridge because they taste delicious, although, like all dried fruit, they are higher in calories than fresh fruit by volume. Porridge is great mood food – it helps to beat stress.

40g porridge oats
200ml skimmed milk
20g goji berries

Put the porridge oats in a bowl. Cover with 180ml milk. Put in the microwave and cook for 1 minute. Stir, then cook for another 1 minute or until creamy, but keep checking – it sometimes needs less time, depending on the quality of your porridge oats and the strength of your microwave. (Alternatively, cook in the traditional way in a pan on the hob. Bring the mixture gently to the boil, then simmer for 5–10 minutes.) Once cooked, add a little more milk, then add the goji berries, and serve.

Blueberry Yoghurt Compote

SERVES 1   CALS: 154

Packed with antioxidants, blueberries are a great way to start your day. The maple syrup in this recipe is on the indulgent side, but I find it really boosts the spirits on a rainy Monday morning. If you want to leave it out, your breakfast will be even healthier.

    100g low-fat or fat-free Greek yoghurt
    1 handful of blueberries (80g)
    1 tsp maple syrup
    2 tsp mixed seeds

Spoon the yoghurt into a bowl, throw on the blueberries, drizzle over the maple syrup and top with the seeds, then serve.

....

Jane Tip ≫ *Try this with dried cranberries instead of mixed seeds, but remember: dried fruit is high in sugar, so you definitely won't need the sweet indulgence of the maple syrup.*

....

Apple, Cinnamon and Walnut Whip

SERVES 1 CALS: 176 with fromage frais; **181** with yoghurt

There's something gorgeously autumnal about this recipe. The sharp sweetness of the apple and the simple smoothness of the fromage frais make it a fast but luxurious breakfast. You may not need the honey, but do add the walnuts to get that protein boost. It will make you feel fuller for longer.

1 apple, sliced
100g fat-free Greek yoghurt or fromage frais
10g walnuts, roughly chopped
1 tsp honey (optional)
a pinch of ground cinnamon

Put the apple in a bowl and add the yoghurt or fromage frais, then stir in the walnuts. Drizzle the honey on top and sprinkle with cinnamon before serving.

QUICK BREAKFAST BUYS

If you really are eating on the run, try these convenient buys:

▶ Grasshopper porridge – ready to go at around 240 calories and available at most supermarkets.

▶ Müller Light yoghurt – available everywhere and only 91 calories.

▶ Pret's Porridge with Cranberry and Pomegranate is 311 calories and their Bircher muesli 304 calories.

LUNCHES

Today, more and more people have busy jobs, so more often than not lunch will be a sandwich eaten hastily at your desk. Others may be at home, but even with the kitchen handy you may not actually sit down for lunch – you're much more likely to be rushing around doing the chores. It's important to take time to lunch, however, and to make sure it is balanced and nutritious. Why? Because if you don't you are more likely to feel hungry later in the afternoon. What's more, up goes the risk of a late-afternoon sugar dip and – especially if your spirits are low – your will may be weak, and that's when the chocolate and cookies start to beckon.

For me, lunch needs to be quick, easy and delicious. I have divided my recipes into two sections: lunches you can eat at your desk, and lunches you can eat at home. They are, however, interchangeable, but the ones you can take to work are slightly simpler to prepare and easier to eat. That said, they also work for a lovely kitchen-table lunch too. There's very little cooking involved in any of these recipes, and they are all either soups or salads. Read on for the reason why.

Why soup? Soup is often listed as an ideal food to include in your diet if you want to lose weight. Eating soup improves satiety – in other words it makes you feel full, so you eat less. It's also a great way to get lots of lovely vegetables into your diet, without having to chomp through an entire plate of greens. It's warming and comforting, and it's generally low in calories. The secret is to enjoy soup without the bread, which is easy if it is tasty and filling, as you will see once you try my recipes.

If you can't make your own soup, most good supermarkets do great ready-made ones in cartons. Just remember the cartons usually serve two – so watch your portion control. You can also get soup 'on the go' now from most popular lunchtime spots – but look at the label to check the calories, and always refuse the bread – even if it's free!

Why salad? I love salads. They are the perfect way to enjoy good food; they are quick and easy to prepare and are full of raw ingredients, bursting with nutrients.

Summer time may be salad time, but salads are not just for the summer – they can be enjoyed whatever the season. Roasted root vegetables and a squeeze of lemon make a fabulous winter salad, a handful of lentils adds substance to a simple green salad on a cold winter's day, while fresh figs bring new life to a salad when the heat has left us as September starts.

One of the best things about salads is that they are very portable. And of course, if you don't have time to make one yourself, you can always pop into a supermarket or lunchtime spot and grab something on the go, but always read the labels to check those calorie counts.

Light lunches – desk-top eating for the working woman

All these lunches are portable. Make the salads in advance and put them into a plastic container, and take the soups in a flask to work. Don't think of them as exclusively for office eating, though; they work equally well at home. Simply make them the night before and you're all set to go in the morning.

Most of the recipes serve more than one person, so freeze extra soup in batches and put additional salad in the fridge to have the following day, or to add to grilled fish or chicken for a simply gorgeous but super-fast supper. Alternatively, you can divide all the recipes by two or four and simply make what you need for your lunch.

Spinach and Rocket Soup

SERVES **4**   CALS: **286** per serving

A glut of green gorgeousness, this soup is guaranteed to take you through the working day without your tummy rumbling.

40g butter
1 tbsp olive oil
1 onion, finely chopped
2 garlic cloves, chopped
350g potatoes, peeled and chopped
1 litre chicken or vegetable stock
1kg fresh spinach, stalks discarded, leaves roughly chopped
250g rocket, roughly chopped
250g low-fat yoghurt
1 tsp freshly grated nutmeg, or to taste
1 handful each of steamed peas and steamed baby leeks, finely sliced
sea salt and freshly ground black pepper

Put the butter, oil and onion into a large pan and fry gently over a medium heat for about 5 minutes. Add the garlic and continue cooking gently for 2 minutes, without colouring. Now add the potatoes and stock. Bring to the boil and simmer gently, uncovered, for 10 minutes or until the potatoes are tender.

Stir in 800g of the spinach and 200g of the rocket. Allow to cool slightly, and then add the remaining spinach and rocket. Pour immediately into a blender and purée. Return the soup to the pan. Add the yoghurt and nutmeg to taste, and then reheat without boiling. Taste, season, and scatter the peas and leeks on the top. Pour into your flask and you're ready to go.

Mushroom and Porcini Soup

SERVES **4** CALS: **227** per serving

This is one of the best-sellers at Jane Plan. Made lovingly in our kitchens, the flavour of the mushrooms combined with the creaminess of the crème fraîche is hard to beat. Mushrooms are a good source of vitamin B and minerals such as selenium, copper and potassium.

25g dried porcini (ceps)
25g butter
25ml olive oil
1 onion, finely chopped
3 garlic cloves, sliced
1 tsp fresh thyme leaves
a splash of white vermouth
400g field mushrooms, any mixture, finely chopped
850ml vegetable stock
200ml low-fat crème fraîche
sea salt and freshly ground black pepper
snipped chives, to serve

Put the dried porcini in a small bowl and pour boiling water over to just cover. Heat the butter and olive oil in a pan over a medium heat, then gently fry the onion, garlic and thyme for 5 minutes until softened and starting to brown. Add a splash of vermouth.

Drain the porcini in a colander, reserving the liquid, then add the porcini to the pan together with the field mushrooms. Leave to cook for 5 minutes until the mushrooms go limp. Pour over the stock and the reserved mushroom liquid and bring to the boil, then simmer for 20 minutes. Add the crème fraîche.

Process the soup using a blender or liquidiser. If you like your soup smooth, pass it through a fine sieve. If you prefer it with mush-roomy bits in, then leave it as it is. Return the blended soup to the pan, add plenty of seasoning and serve with snipped chives on top.

Carrot and Coriander Soup

SERVES 4   **CALS: 135** per serving

This ever-popular soup is silky and smooth, sweet and simply delicious. Crammed full of vitamin A, the benefits of carrots go far beyond just being good for your eyesight.

> 1 small knob of butter, the size of the tip of your thumb or
> 1 tbsp olive oil (the butter makes a smoother, silkier soup)
> 1 onion, chopped
> 1 tsp ground coriander
> 1 medium potato, chopped
> 450g carrots, chopped
> 1.2 litres vegetable or chicken stock
> 1 handful of fresh coriander leaves, finely chopped
> 4 tbsp half-fat crème fraîche
> sea salt and freshly ground black pepper

Heat the butter in a large pan, add the onion and fry for 5 minutes until softened. Stir in the ground coriander and potato, and cook for 1 minute. Add the carrots and stock, then bring to the boil and reduce the heat. Cover and simmer for 20 minutes or until the carrots are tender.

Pour into a blender with the fresh coriander and blitz until smooth (you may need to do this in two batches). Return to the pan, taste and adjust the seasoning, then reheat and stir in the crème fraîche. Serve or pour into your flask to take to work.

Red Lentil, Chickpea and Chilli Soup

SERVES **4**   CALS: **343** per serving

This is a bowl of beany goodness (or a flask of fat-free fabulousness). Eating a warming, beany soup at lunchtime will help you avoid that late-afternoon sugar dip and keep you concentrating until it's time to go home.

- 2 tsp cumin seeds
- 1 tbsp olive oil
- 2 garlic cloves
- 3 large shallots
- 1 large red chilli, deseeded and finely sliced
- 140g split red lentils
- 850ml chicken stock
- 400g can chopped tomatoes
- 200g canned chickpeas, rinsed and drained
- a small handful of fresh coriander leaves, chopped, plus extra leaves to serve
- 4 tbsp low-fat crème fraîche or low-fat/fat-free Greek yoghurt
- sea salt and freshly ground black pepper

Heat a large pan over a medium heat and dry-fry the cumin seeds for 1 minute, or until they start to pop and release their aromas. Add the oil, garlic, shallots and chilli (holding back a few slices for later), and cook for 5 minutes. Stir in the lentils, stock and tomatoes, then bring to the boil. Simmer for 15 minutes or until the lentils have softened.

Whiz the soup with a blender or food processor until it forms a rough purée, then pour back into the pan and add the chickpeas. Heat gently, then season well and stir in the chopped coriander. Finish with a dollop of crème fraîche and sprinkle with coriander leaves and the remaining sliced chilli. Now pour into your flask. (If serving at the table, add the crème fraîche, coriander and chilli to each individual bowl.)

· ·

Jane Tip » *This soup is higher in calories than most. Think hard about your supper choice if you have this for lunch, and make sure you have enough calorie credit left.*

· ·

ESSENTIAL PROTEIN

Protein keeps you feeling fuller for longer, so if, for example, you opt for a vegetable soup for lunch and still feel a tad peckish, choose a protein-rich snack from the snack list on pages 146–8. A hard-boiled egg, a handful of nuts or some yoghurt are all good choices.

Summer Soup

SERVES **4**   CALS: **192** per serving

I call this Summer Soup because it uses the vegetables I most asso-
ciate with the warmer months: broad beans, peas and courgettes.
However, I recommend frozen peas and beans, because I like to
make it all year round and they are so much more accessible and
quicker to use – and I'm convenience girl! But come early summer,
when the peas and broad beans are sweet and bursting with goodness, find some time to do some podding and enjoy the taste of
sunshine in your soup. Use a good-quality shop-bought pesto if
you don't have time to make your own.

    1 tbsp olive oil, plus a little extra for the pesto
    1 leek, finely chopped
    1 garlic clove, sliced
    500g courgettes, quartered lengthways and chopped
    400g frozen broad beans
    200g frozen peas
    1 litre hot vegetable stock
    1 handful of pine nuts
    1 tbsp grated pecorino cheese
    1 handful of basil leaves, torn into small pieces

Heat the oil in a large pan over a medium heat. Cook the leek and
garlic for a few seconds, then add the courgettes and broad beans
and cook for 3 minutes or until they start to soften. Stir in the peas,
pour on the hot stock and cook for a further 3 minutes or until all
the vegetables are cooked through.

Using a pestle and mortar, grind the pine nuts, pecorino, basil
and a small slug of olive oil into a soft pesto paste and stir through
the soup. It's flask-ready now!

Spicy Butternut Squash and Pumpkin Soup

SERVES 4   **CALS: 190** per serving

There's nothing more annoying than having half a butternut squash and half a pumpkin left over, so I usually double up here and make twice the amount. It freezes really well.

½ butternut squash, peeled and cubed
½ small pumpkin, peeled and cubed
2 tbsp olive oil
1 onion, finely chopped
2 carrots, sliced
2 celery sticks, finely sliced
1 garlic clove, crushed
1 tsp curry powder
1.25 litres vegetable stock
150ml low-fat crème fraîche
1 tbsp pumpkin seeds
fresh thyme leaves, to serve
sea salt and freshly ground black pepper

Preheat the oven to 200°C/Gas 6. Put the butternut squash and pumpkin in a roasting tin, drizzle over 1 tbsp of the oil and season. Roast for 25–30 minutes until golden brown, turning occasionally.

Put the onion in a large pan over a medium heat with the remaining oil and add the carrots, celery and garlic with the curry powder. Cook for 4–5 minutes until softened.

Add the roasted butternut squash and pumpkin to the pan, then pour over the vegetable stock. Bring to the boil, then cover and simmer for 20–30 minutes until all the vegetables are tender.

Purée the soup in a food processor until smooth. Season with salt and pepper.

Transfer the soup to a clean pan and stir in the crème fraîche. Serve in warm bowls and sprinkle with pumpkin seeds and some thyme leaves.

Haricot Bean Soup

SERVES **6**   CALS: **175** per serving

This is about as simple as soup can be. Had a hard day at work? Simply put all the ingredients into a pan, simmer for an hour (while you shower, watch the TV or relax) and it will be ready to pour into your flask.

2 litres vegetable stock
400g can haricot beans, drained and rinsed
2 carrots, chopped
1 large onion, chopped
1 celery stick, chopped
1 bay leaf
a dash of Tabasco sauce, to taste (optional)
sea salt and freshly ground black pepper

Put the stock in a pan over a medium heat and add the beans. Heat gently, then add the carrots, onion, celery and bay leaf. Cook for 1 hour or until the vegetables are tender. Remove the bay leaf. Season with salt and pepper and serve with Tabasco, if you like.

Jane Tip » *This soup is chunky, so rather than trying to drink it from your flask, pour it into a bowl (keep one handy at work).*

Classic Crudités

SERVES **1** CALS: **232** with hummus; **124** with reduced-fat cottage cheese; **121** with tzatziki

I have made this into a recipe for one, because it is the perfect desk lunch if you are super-busy, and making it just for yourself takes only a couple of minutes. You can cut up the crudités while the kettle boils in the morning, put them into a plastic bag or box and you're ready to go.

> 2 large handfuls of your favourite vegetables, such as carrots, cucumber, celery, radishes, baby tomatoes, baby corn, mangetouts or French beans
> 300g low-fat hummus, cottage cheese or tzatziki

Cut the carrots, cucumber and celery into large matchsticks (other suggested vegetables can remain whole). Put into a plastic container or a plastic bag ready to take.

When it comes to lunch, put your crudités and one-third of your chosen pot of hummus, cottage cheese or tzatziki onto a plate. Start dipping.

....

Jane Tip » *Don't be tempted to dip from the pot – you'll eat more than a third. If you want to add extra substance, an oatcake is about 42 calories.*

....

Rocket and Parma Ham Twists

SERVES 2 (makes 4 twists per person)   **CALS: 150** per serving

Combine this fun finger lunch with the crudités idea on the previous page. I often make this at my desk. At lunchtime I whiz out and buy a packet of Parma ham and a bag of rocket, then get rolling. It's nice to add the poppy seeds or black pepper, but as every working woman knows, sometimes you just have to make do. And they taste equally delicious without the added extras.

> 1 bag of long-stemmed wild rocket
> 8 slices of Parma ham
> black poppy seeds (if you can find them) or freshly ground
>   black pepper

Take a small handful of rocket. Make sure the stems are at one end and the leafy parts at the other. Wrap a piece of Parma ham around them. Sprinkle with seeds or pepper.

....

Jane Tip » *For variety, try using smoked salmon slices instead of Parma ham, and add a squeeze of lemon.*

These twists also make great pre-dinner nibbles if you are entertaining, and are fabulous for picnics.

....

Celery, Manchego and Almond Salad with Quince Jelly

SERVES **4**   CALS: **279** per serving

Wonderful in winter, this is a gourmet treat. The protein from the almonds combined with the fibre from the celery make this a crunchy, munchy, filling salad. Best of all, celery is supposed to have negative calories – the energy used to digest it outweighs the calories in the celery itself.

  8 celery sticks
  200g Manchego cheese, thinly shaved
  40g almonds
  a splash of olive oil
  4 tsp quince jelly
  sea salt

Thinly slice the celery sticks on the diagonal and put into a bowl. Add the Manchego and almonds, and toss together.

  Before leaving for work in the morning add the olive oil and sea salt to the bowl and toss the salad. Then put it in your container, with the quince jelly on the top. If serving at home, toss all the ingredients and put the tossed salad onto a plate with the quince jelly on the side, so that everyone can help themselves.

....

Jane Tip » *This salad works equally well with Stilton, walnuts and mango chutney instead of the Manchego, almonds and quince jelly.*

....

Salmon and Rocket Salad with Horseradish

SERVES **4**   CALS: **180** per serving

This salad is a firm favourite. It can be made in minutes, tastes utterly delicious and is full of iron. If you're in a rush, don't worry about grating the lemon zest or adding the crème fraîche. It's still gorgeous without.

> 4 generous handfuls of wild rocket
> 400g smoked salmon slices
> 2 tbsp horseradish
> 2 tbsp half-fat crème fraîche
> 2 gherkins, chopped
> 1 lemon
> dill sprigs, to garnish

Put the rocket at the bottom of your container. Roll up the slices of smoked salmon and arrange them on the top. Mix the horseradish, crème fraîche and chopped gherkins together in a bowl and leave to one side.

In the morning before you leave for work, grate the lemon zest on top of the salmon and squeeze the lemon juice over the salad, then add a spoonful of the horseradish mixture. Finish with a sprig of dill.

If serving at the table, put the rocket on a plate, add the rolled smoked salmon, zest and squeeze the lemon and put the horse-radish in a bowl so that everyone can help themselves. Garnish your salad with dill, then serve.

Quinoa, Crudités and Parmesan Salad

SERVES **4**   CALS: **349** per serving

I love this salad. Bringing together the power of protein with the vitamins, minerals and fibre from a variety of gorgeous raw veggies it can be rightly called a super-food salad.

170g quinoa
35g pine nuts
300g baby asparagus, sugar snaps and carrot sticks
   (or any other crudités you fancy)
225g chicory, finely sliced on the diagonal
55g Parmesan cheese, shaved
4 tbsp olive oil
juice of 1 lemon
sea salt

Cook the quinoa according to the pack instructions and leave to cool. Meanwhile, toast the pine nuts in a dry frying pan over a medium-high heat for 4–6 minutes, then transfer to a plate to cool.

Combine the quinoa, pine nuts, crudités, chicory and Parmesan in a bowl.

The next morning, add the olive oil, lemon juice and salt, and toss together, then put everything in your sealable container. If eating at home, toss the salad with the olive oil, lemon juice and salt just before serving.

Fig, Fennel and Parma Ham Salad

SERVES 4   CALS: 154 per serving

Ripe figs and aniseedy fennel are a marriage made in heaven. Figs are sweet, jammy and oozing with flavour, whereas in contrast fennel is sharp and pungent. Full of phytonutrients, fennel can add punch to any green salad, but in this recipe it has a starring role.

    2 fennel bulbs, finely sliced
    3 tbsp snipped chives
    2 tbsp olive oil
    a pinch of sea salt
    zest and juice of 1 lemon
    12 slices of Parma ham
    8 figs, halved

Put the fennel in a large bowl, then add the chives, oil, salt, lemon zest and juice. Toss and leave to stand (you can leave it overnight in the fridge).

Just before you leave for work, put 3 slices of Parma ham in your container, put 2 figs on top, then scatter the fennel salad over them. If serving at home, divide the Parma ham between the serving plates, put the figs on top then scatter the fennel salad on top.

....

Jane Tip » *If your calorie budget allows, you can add mozzarella to this salad too. Use a whole ball (usually about 125g) and budget for an additional 87 calories per person, assuming you each have a quarter of the mozzarella ball.*

....

Smoked Mackerel and Watercress with Orange Salad

SERVES **4**   CALS: **250** per serving

The fresh zesty oranges and the full flavour of the red onions complement the deep, strong flavours of the mackerel here. Adding the mackerel means you'll be getting plenty of omega-3 fatty acids, which are great for the health of your heart.

2 large oranges
¼ red onion, very finely sliced
2 tsp white wine vinegar
2 tsp olive oil
1 fresh chilli, deseeded and finely chopped
a small handful of fresh thyme leaves
4 fillets of smoked mackerel (about 50g each – check the
   packaging to ensure yours is this size)
4 handfuls of watercress
4 tsp horseradish
sea salt

Using a sharp knife, cut a thin slice of peel and pith from each end of an orange. Put cut-side down on a plate and cut off the peel and pith in strips. Remove any remaining pith. Cut into slices. Repeat with the other orange.

Arrange the orange and red onion slices on a plate. Drizzle over the vinegar and olive oil. Scatter over the chilli and thyme leaves, then sprinkle over some salt – but be careful, mackerel is quite salty already. Put the mackerel on top. Add a generous handful of watercress on the side and 1 tsp horseradish to each serving. When you're ready to leave for work, put the whole lot in your container.

Kitchen-table lunches — weekend eating for friends and family

The lunch recipes that follow are perfect for Saturday and Sunday lunches but are also great if you're home alone during the week. Most of them are for four or two people and work well for weekend entertaining or family eating, but if you're home alone, you can either divide the quantities into individual servings or freeze one-portion sizes. Most of the soups freeze really well, or will keep in the fridge overnight, ready for lunch the following day. Many of the salads will also keep in the fridge overnight, but add the dressings just before serving, otherwise the salad may go soggy.

Jane Wisdom

If you are home alone, make sure you don't make enough for four and then eat for four! Portion control is the key to success on Jane Plan. Serve yourself and put the leftovers away – straight away.

Tom Yum Soup

SERVES **2** CALS: **90** per serving

Quick, easy and delicious, this soup will fill your kitchen with aromas from the East. And it's deliciously low in calories too – great if you're planning to eat a more indulgent dinner later in the day and need to keep some calories in the bank. Alternatively, serve this on a Sunday evening, if you've had a special lunch.

700ml chicken stock, or use water and a stock cube
1 lemongrass stalk, outer leaves removed, sliced into pieces
5 thick slices of peeled ginger
8 fresh coriander stems, leaves separated and stems chopped
3 fresh or frozen kaffir lime leaves, finely chopped
2 large handfuls of prawns (for ease and convenience, I use frozen peeled prawns)
3 tbsp fish sauce
6 green and red bird's eye chillies, deseeded and chopped
4 tbsp lime juice
1 handful of mint leaves, finely chopped

Bring the stock to the boil in a medium pan. Add the lemongrass, ginger, coriander stems and lime leaves, then simmer for 2 minutes. Add the prawns, fish sauce, chillies and lime juice, then return to the boil. Taste and adjust the seasoning with either more lime juice or fish sauce. Top with the coriander leaves and finely chopped mint before serving.

Moroccan Chickpea Soup with Harissa

SERVES **4**   CALS: **159** per serving

Hot, spicy and filling, this soup is good served with flatbread, yoghurt, hummus and a bowl of spicy black olives, so your hungry family (and anyone else not calorie counting) can dig into the extras! That said, the soup is so satisfying on its own that you won't feel deprived. I have included optional honey. Moroccan food is traditionally often sweet, but I think this recipe works just as well without the sweetness.

1 tbsp olive oil

1 onion, chopped

2 garlic cloves, finely chopped

1 tsp ground cumin

1 red chilli, deseeded and roughly chopped

2cm fresh root ginger, peeled and grated

1 tsp ras-el-hanout

¼ tsp cinnamon

600ml vegetable or chicken stock

400g can chopped plum tomatoes

400g can chickpeas, rinsed and drained

100g frozen broad beans

zest and juice of 1 lemon

honey, to taste (optional)

1½ tsp harissa paste, or to taste

1 large handful of fresh coriander and mint leaves, finely chopped

sea salt and freshly ground black pepper

Heat the oil in a large pan over a medium-low heat, then fry the onion gently for 10 minutes until softened, but not browned. Tip in the garlic, cumin, chilli, ginger, ras-el-hanout and cinnamon, and fry for another 1 minute. Add the stock and tomatoes, plus a good grind of black pepper. Simmer, covered, for 8 minutes.

Using a blender or food processor, purée until smooth, then return to the pan, adding more liquid if needed. Add the chickpeas and cook for a further 3 minutes or until the chickpeas are warmed through, then add the broad beans and cook until tender. Add the lemon juice.

Add some honey, but taste the soup first; I often prefer the sharp taste of the soup without the honey, it depends on my mood. Season to taste, then top with a sprinkling of lemon zest, the harissa and chopped herbs, and serve.

....

Jane Tip >> *This is quick and easy to make, because it uses mainly store-cupboard ingredients. I have suggested it as a kitchen-table lunch, because it's very chunky and would be hard to drink from a flask. Also, adding the fresh herbs at the end really lifts it, and they would lose their oomph if left warm in a flask. That said, it is portable – so do make in advance and take to work if you want to.*

....

Thai Fish Soup

SERVES **2**   CALS: **182** per serving

    500ml chicken or fish stock
    1 tbsp Thai red curry paste
    4 fresh or frozen kaffir lime leaves
    1 tbsp fish sauce
    200g skinless cod or swordfish, cut into 3cm cubes
    80g broccoli florets
    100g raw king prawns
    2 pak choi, leaves separated
    juice of ½ lime
    1 handful of fresh coriander leaves
    1 red bird's eye chilli, deseeded and chopped

Put the stock in a large pan and stir in the curry paste, lime leaves, fish sauce and 250ml water. Bring to the boil then reduce to a simmer and cook for 5 minutes. Add the fish and broccoli to the pan. Simmer for 2 minutes, uncovered.

Stir in the prawns, pak choi and the lime juice, and simmer for another 2–3 minutes or until the fish and prawns are just cooked. Serve in bowls scattered with coriander and chilli.

••

Jane Tip » *If you have a hungry partner or child expecting something more substantial, boil some noodles in a separate pan. Once cooked, drain and put them on their plate, then serve the Thai Fish Soup poured over the noodles. You can enjoy yours without the noodles – equally delicious but with half the calories.*

••

Pea and Mint Soup

SERVES 4 **CALS: 183** per serving

Clean eating at its best. I love the fresh flavours in this summery soup.

  1 tbsp olive oil
  1 small knob of butter, no bigger than the tip of your thumb
  1 bunch of spring onions, roughly chopped
  1 medium potato, peeled and diced
  1 garlic clove, crushed
  850ml vegetable or chicken stock
  400g frozen peas (or 900g fresh peas in the pod, shelled)
  4 tbsp chopped fresh mint leaves, plus extra mint leaves
    to serve
  1 tbsp fresh lemon or lime juice
  150ml half-fat crème fraîche, plus extra to serve
  sea salt and freshly ground black pepper

Heat the oil and butter in a pan over a medium heat. Add the spring onions, potato and garlic, and gently fry for a few minutes, without colouring. Add the stock. Bring to the boil, then reduce the heat and simmer for 15 minutes or until the potato is very soft. Add the peas and simmer for 5 minutes.

Stir in the mint and lemon juice. Cool slightly, then blend using a liquidiser or food processor until smooth. Stir in the crème fraîche, then taste and season with salt and pepper.

To serve the soup cold, cool the soup and chill it – you may need to add more stock to the soup before serving it, as it will thicken as it cools. To serve hot, return the soup to the rinsed-out pan and reheat gently, without boiling. Top each bowl with a fresh mint leaf and 1 tsp of crème fraîche.

Zesty Carrot and Orange Soup

SERVES **6**   CALS: **183** per serving

This classic combination will give you a real blast of vitamin C.

25g butter
225g onions, sliced
700g carrots, sliced
1 litre chicken or vegetable stock
1 large sweet orange, such as a blood orange
2 tbsp low-fat crème fraîche
1 handful of pumpkin seeds
fresh coriander leaves, chopped
sea salt and freshly ground black pepper

Melt the butter in a pan over a medium heat. Add the onions and carrots, and cook gently for 10 minutes or until slightly softened. Add the stock and bring to the boil. Lower the heat, cover and simmer for about 40 minutes, or until the vegetables are tender.

Using a blender or food processor, purée the vegetables and the stock. Return the soup to the pan and finely grate half the orange zest into the soup. Stir well to combine with the ingredients in the pan. Squeeze the orange juice into the pan. Reheat the soup gently, then taste and adjust the seasoning. Serve in bowls topped with a dollop of crème fraîche and a sprinkle of pumpkin seeds and chopped coriander.

....

Jane Tip » *Hot crusty bread is a lovely accompaniment for the non-dieters, but don't be tempted yourself. It tastes delicious without the added extras.*

....

Thai Chicken and Courgette Soup

SERVES **2**   CALS: **180** per serving

This recipe makes enough soup for you to come back for seconds. You've probably noticed by now that I'm very keen on Thai soups. I find that when eating an Asian spicy soup I am less likely to hanker after a piece of crusty bread or some hot buttered toast. What's more, it is said that eating chilli can suppress the appetite, so not only will you find that these soups taste delicious but you will also feel completely satisfied. What more could anyone ask for?

1 litre chicken stock
1 tbsp Thai red or green curry paste
1 tbsp fish sauce, plus extra to serve
2 tsp sugar, plus extra to serve
zest and juice of 2 limes, plus extra juice to serve
100g courgettes, sliced
1 bunch of spring onions, sliced, white and the green parts separated
200g leftover cooked chicken, shredded, or two small chicken breasts, cooked and cut into thin slices
1 handful of fresh coriander leaves
1 red bird's eye chilli, deseeded and chopped

Pour the stock into a pan, then stir in the curry paste, fish sauce, sugar, lime juice and most of the zest. Bring to the boil, then add the courgettes and the spring onion whites. Cover, and simmer for 2 minutes. Stir in the chicken and add the spring onion greens, then gently heat through.

Serve in bowls scattered with the remaining lime zest, the coriander leaves and chopped chilli. Put extra lime juice, sugar and fish sauce on the side so that everyone can help themselves and adjust the flavour to their taste.

Watercress Soup

SERVES **6**   CALS: **202** per serving

This is an all-time classic, and even without cream it tastes good. Adding the yoghurt at the end is essential, as it gives it added sharpness. If you decide to make this at home to take to work, simply reheat the soup, add the yoghurt and then fill your flask.

50g butter
3 tbsp olive oil
3–4 banana shallots (or a large onion), chopped
2 bunches of watercress
50g plain flour
750ml chicken or vegetable stock
300ml semi-skimmed milk
2 tbsp low-fat yoghurt
sea salt and freshly ground black pepper

Melt the butter and oil in a pan over a medium heat, add the shallots and cook gently for 10 minutes or until soft but not coloured. Meanwhile, trim the watercress, leaving some of the stem (keeping a little of the stem enhances the flavour), put 6 sprigs aside then roughly chop the remainder. Add the chopped watercress to the shallots. Cover the pan with a lid and cook gently for a further 4 minutes.

Add the flour and cook gently, stirring, for 1–2 minutes. Remove from the heat and gradually blend in the stock and milk. Bring to the boil, stirring constantly, then simmer for 3 minutes. Season to taste.

Purée the soup in a blender or food processor. Return to the rinsed-out pan and reheat gently, without boiling. Taste and adjust the seasoning, if needed. Serve in individual bowls and add a dollop of yoghurt on top of each bowl and a sprig of watercress.

Warm Halloumi Salad with Chilli Dressing

SERVES **4**   CALS: **383** per serving

3 ripe peaches or nectarines, halved and stoned
250g halloumi cheese
2 tbsp groundnut oil
3 red or white chicory hearts, quartered lengthways
1 bunch of spring onions, sliced diagonally
mixed salad leaves, to serve
mint sprig, to garnish

For the dressing

1 red chilli, deseeded and finely chopped
1 handful of fresh mint leaves, finely chopped
1 handful of fresh coriander leaves, roughly chopped
juice of 2 lemons
2 tbsp clear honey

To make the dressing, put the chilli in a small jug and add the mint, coriander, lemon juice and honey. Stir well to combine, then leave to one side.

Cut each peach half into five wedges. Pat the cheese dry on kitchen paper, then cut into thin slices.

Heat 1 tbsp of the oil in a large frying pan and fry the cheese for 30 seconds on each side, until lightly coloured. Add the chicory and onions, and fry quickly over a high heat. Remove from the pan. Heat the remaining oil in the pan and add the peach wedges, then fry for 30 seconds on each side.

Put the salad leaves on a serving platter and put the peaches, cheese, onions and chicory on the top. Finally, drizzle the chilli dressing over the salad and top with a sprig of mint.

Warm Hummus with Chilli Flakes and Infused Olive Oil

SERVES 4 **CALS: 409** per serving

My friend Ozlem, founder of Ozlem's Turkish Table, a cookery school based in Surrey, gave this delicious recipe to me. Interestingly, in Turkey, hummus is traditionally eaten warm, so I've made it a kitchen-table treat.

225g dried chickpeas, soaked in water overnight, or
   3 x 400g cans chickpeas, rinsed and drained
4 tbsp extra virgin olive oil, plus extra if needed
juice of 1 lemon
1–2 garlic cloves, to taste, crushed (optional)
1–2 tbsp tahini, to taste
1 tsp salt, or to taste
1 tsp ground cumin, or to taste

To serve
2 tbsp olive oil
½ tsp dried chilli flakes or paprika
½ tsp ground cumin (optional)

If using dried chickpeas, drain the chickpeas and transfer them to a pan. Cover well with cold water. Bring to the boil and boil for 10 minutes, then lower the heat and partially cover the pan. Simmer the chickpeas for 1 hour or until they are soft and easy to mash.

Put the chickpeas in a food processor and add the oil, 2 tbsp water, the lemon juice, garlic and tahini. Blend until fairly smooth. If the mixture becomes thick and difficult to blend, add a little more olive oil or water. Season with salt, and stir in the cumin. Process until you have a soft, smooth paste. Chill until required.

Just before serving, warm the hummus in a pan for a couple of minutes. In a separate pan, heat the olive oil over a medium-low heat and stir in the chilli flakes. Combine for a minute or two to allow the chilli flakes to infuse the olive oil. Put the warm hummus on a plate and drizzle the chilli-infused olive oil over the top. You can sprinkle some extra ground cumin over the top, if you like, before serving.

Jane Tip » *You may be surprised to see just how many calories there are in this dish, so serve with crudités rather than pitta bread!*

Jane Wisdom

Chickpeas are a good source of fibre, which can help keep cholesterol levels low and promote better heart health. Fibre-rich chickpeas can also help people with diabetes keep a check on their blood sugar levels.

Grilled Vegetables with Goat's Cheese Salad

SERVES **4** CALS: **254** per serving

Not just for lunch – on hot, steamy days, this works equally well for dinner.

  a bunch of baby asparagus spears
  250g broad beans
  1 tbsp olive oil
  1 large red onion, halved and thinly sliced
  150g baby mushrooms
  250g baby courgettes, halved lengthways
  120ml fat-free crème fraîche
  a small bunch of dill leaves, roughly chopped
  zest of 2 lemons and juice of 1
  150g goat's cheese, cut into 1cm slices
  sea salt and freshly ground black pepper

Snap off any woody ends from the asparagus stalks at the point where they break easily and discard. Put the asparagus and broad beans in boiling water and blanch for 3 minutes, then drain in a colander.

Heat the oil in a pan over a medium heat and gently fry the onion, mushrooms and courgettes for 8–10 minutes. Add the asparagus, crème fraîche, half the dill, the lemon zest and juice. Cook, stirring, for 2 minutes. Season and sprinkle the remaining dill on top. Preheat the grill, then lightly grease an ovenproof dish and spoon in the mixture.

Put the goat's cheese on top of the vegetables and put under the grill until the cheese is melting and beginning to brown. Serve.

Butternut and Beetroot Salad

SERVES 4 CALS: 219 per serving without the dressing;
256 per serving with the dressing

Wonderful in winter, and sensational in summer, this year-round salad ticks all the boxes. The mellowness of the butternut squash, the sweetness of the beetroot and the sharpness of the feta make this one of my favourites. Beetroot is brilliant in so many ways – if you don't have time to make this salad, a plate of beetroot, a teaspoon of horseradish and a sprinkle of sea salt makes a great light lunch when the pressure is on.

½ large butternut squash, peeled and sliced into 5mm discs
a pinch of dried chilli flakes
1 tbsp olive oil
2 large ready-cooked beetroots (without vinegar), sliced
  into circles
2 tbsp pine nuts
150g feta cheese, crumbled
a small handful of fresh mint leaves, finely chopped
sea salt and freshly ground black pepper

For the dressing
1 tbsp pomegranate seeds
½ tbsp lemon juice
2 tbsp extra virgin olive oil

Heat the oven to 200°C/Gas 6. Lay the squash in a roasting tin. Scatter the chilli on top, season well, drizzle with the oil and roast for 20–25 minutes, turning halfway through.

Remove from the oven and pile onto a plate, with the beetroot. Sprinkle over the pine nuts, feta cheese and chopped mint.

To make the dressing, put all the ingredients in a screwtop jar and give it a good shake, then drizzle the dressing over the top of the salad before serving.

....

Jane Tip » *When buying butternut squash go for unblemished fruit that feels heavy for its size, with a matt rather than glossy skin. A shiny one can mean that it has been picked too early so it won't be as sweet as a fully-grown one.*

....

Jane Wisdom

Research suggests that beetroot lowers blood pressure, so if yours is high or life is stressful, don't hold back.

Watermelon Salad with Feta and Pine Nuts

SERVES **4**   CALS: **300** per serving

Refreshingly delicious – this salad is one of my favourites. While researching this recipe I came across all kinds of watermelon facts: it can ease sore muscles (great if you like a hard workout); it helps boost circulation; and it is apparently a natural Viagra too (although you'd have to eat an awful lot of it). Whatever your reason for enjoying watermelon, rest assured that it is rich in vitamins A and C.

    350g watermelon, cut into small chunks
    250g feta cheese, cubed
    20 pitted black olives
    200g wild rocket
    4 tbsp fresh mint leaves, roughly chopped
    3 tbsp olive oil
    1 tbsp balsamic vinegar
    1 tbsp lemon juice
    2 tsp pine nuts

Put the watermelon in a large bowl and add the feta cheese. Scatter the olives and the rocket over the top and stir gently to combine.

Put all the remaining ingredients (except the pine nuts) into a screwtop jar and shake to combine. Drizzle over the salad, then scatter the pine nuts over the top.

Jane Tip » *Try to get wild rocket if you can for its peppery flavour.*

Salmon, Broad Beans, Lime, Mint and Ricotta

SERVES 2 CALS: **280** per serving for the salad;
470 per serving with grilled fillet of salmon

This recipe is my flexible friend. I love it for a casual light lunch without the salmon, but a fillet of grilled salmon gives it a boost.

    4 salmon fillets, about 175g each
    3 tbsp olive oil, plus extra for brushing
    300g frozen broad beans
    zest and juice of 1 lime
    1 handful of fresh mint leaves, finely chopped
    80g ricotta cheese
    sea salt and freshly ground black pepper

Preheat the grill to medium-high. Put the salmon fillets on a grill rack and lightly brush with oil. Grill for 15–20 minutes until cooked through.

Meanwhile, put the broad beans in a pan and add water to cover. Bring to the boil then simmer for 5 minutes or until tender. Drain in a colander, then refresh under cold water, and drain again. Put them in a bowl and add the lime zest and juice, the mint and olive oil. Season to taste, then crumble the ricotta over the top. Serve the salmon on top of the salad.

Tomato and Sea Bass Ceviche

SERVES **4** CALS: **205** per serving

I first ate ceviche when I was on my 'big diet' 22 years ago. I was in a restaurant, staring at the menu not knowing what to order. (I was desperate not to break my diet). Then I saw ceviche. I had no idea what it was, so I asked the waiter – it sounded perfect, and it was!

800g tomatoes, cut into small pieces
500g very fresh sea bass, very thinly sliced
50g fresh coriander leaves, chopped
1 red chilli, finely sliced
½ red onion, finely sliced
½ garlic clove, crushed
zest and juice of 2 limes
a dash of olive oil
sea salt and freshly ground black pepper
mixed green salad, to serve

Put the tomatoes and sea bass slices in a bowl, then add the coriander, chilli, onion and garlic.

Add the lime zest and juice to the mixture and leave to marinate for 1½ hours. Season and add a dash of olive oil. Serve on a platter with lots of green leaves.

....

Jane Tip » *Add couscous with chopped cucumber and parsley for non-dieters.*

....

Warm Asparagus Niçoise

SERVES **2**   CALS: **254** per serving

For a lover of seasonal cooking, there's nothing quite like the first crop of asparagus to herald the beginning of spring. Forget the concept of slathering it with butter – instead think fresh and clean. Treat asparagus spears with care – barely show them the heat and they will stay tender and succulent. Think fast cooking but slow eating.

4 radishes, thinly sliced
1 tbsp olive oil, plus extra for drizzling
4 medium free-range eggs, hard-boiled
16 asparagus spears
2 tbsp finely chopped chives
1 tbsp capers, rinsed and chopped
1 tbsp pitted black olives, chopped
1 small chilli, deseeded and finely chopped
sea salt and freshly ground black pepper

Put the radishes in a bowl, add the olive oil and season with salt and pepper, then toss together. Peel and chop the eggs.

Snap off any woody ends from the asparagus stalks at the point where they break easily and discard. Steam the asparagus, then transfer to a bowl, and add a drizzle of olive oil and a pinch of salt.

Scatter the warm asparagus over a plate and top with the radishes, egg, chives, capers and olives. Sprinkle over the chopped chilli and serve.

· ·

Jane Tip » *Asparagus has around 20 calories per 100g, making this recipe a great take on a classic Niçoise salad.*

· ·

ON THE HIGH STREET ...

I know how hard it can be sometimes to plan and prepare lunch. Whether you are working or not, time is tight for us all. On those stressful, busy days, when life is a whirl, check out what the high street has to offer at lunchtime. To give you an idea of the sort of thing to look out for, here are some of my current favourites (in no particular order) . Beware, however, recipes – and hence calorie counts – do change, so be label savvy and check the calories before you buy.

Boots (look for their Shapers range)

▶ Around the World Oriental-style King Prawn, Mango and Sweet Fire Chilli Wrap – 267 calories

▶ Barbecue Chicken Wrap – 294 calories

▶ Chicken Caesar Salad – 205 calories

▶ Tuna and Cucumber Sandwich – 293 calories

▶ Wholesome Egg, Radish and Salad Cream Sandwich – 294 calories

▶ Hummus and Falafel Wrap – 292 calories

▶ Wholesome Goats Cheese and Red Quinoa Salad – 210 calories

▶ Chicken Fajita Pasta Salad – 307 calories

▶ King Prawn and Smoked Salmon Sandwich – 316 calories

→

Marks & Spencer

► Count On Us Chicken and Bacon Caesar Pasta Salad – 110 calories per 100g

► Count On Us Nacho Chicken Wrap – 275 calories per pack

► Count On Us Roasted Butternut Squash with Red Pepper Hummus Wrap – 245 calories per pack

► Count On Us Smoked Turkey and Ham Bagel – 280 calories

Prêt a Manger

► Butternut Squash and Sage Soup – 104 calories

► Chef's Italian Chicken Salad – 306 calories (undressed)

► Roasted Veg and Feta Salad – 195 calories (undressed)

► Chicken, Edamame and Ginger Soup – 137 calories

► Tuna Niçoise Salad – 168 calories (undressed)

Starbucks

► Half-fat Cheddar with Tomato and Apple Chutney Sandwich – 299 calories

► Low-fat Ham and Soft Cheese Sandwich – 297 calories

► Lightly Spiced Chicken Sandwich – 287 calories

Tesco

► Thai Green Curry Soup (have half a carton) – 210 calories per serving

→

▸ Chunky Minestrone Soup (have half a carton) –
150 calories per serving

▸ Prawn, Tuna and Vegetable Sushi – 215 calories

Waitrose

▸ Taiko Sushi Vegetable Sushi – 200 calories per pack

▸ Taiko Sushi Vegetarian Wrap – 120 calories per 100g

▸ Taiko Sushi Brown Rice Nigiri – 221 calories per pack

▸ Taiko Simple Tuna Sushi Wrap – 178 calories

▸ Taiko Sushi Salmon Wrap – 153 calories

▸ Good to Go Rare Beef and Horseradish Sauce Sandwich –
322 calories

▸ Love Life Tuna and Cucumber Sandwich – 321 calories

▸ Good to Go Salmon and Cucumber Sandwich –
333 calories

Miscellaneous

▸ New Covent Garden British Chicken and Ham Soup (have
half a carton) – 186 calories per serving

▸ New Covent Garden Skinny Tomato and Vegetable Green
Soup (have half a carton) – 154 calories per serving

▸ Innocent Veg Pot Thai Coconut Curry – 240 calories

▸ Innocent Rendang Noodle Pot – 266 calories

▸ Innocent Veg Pot Mexican Chilli – 332 calories

DINNERS

After a long hard day, dinner is something to look forward to. It needs to be totally delicious, but also as quick and convenient as possible, allowing you maximum relaxation time. Many of you will be wondering how on earth you are going to squeeze cooking dinner into your already hectic life. Knowing how you feel, I have tried to make these recipes super-quick to prepare, often using store-cupboard ingredients or food from the freezer. No trooping around the supermarket looking for those elusive hard-to-find ingredients.

I have divided my dinners into two sections: Thinner Dinners, which are healthy recipes for every day, with fewer than 450 calories per serving; and Sinner Dinners, which you can use when you feel like a treat or have had a very light lunch and plenty of saved calories in the bank!

I also know how hard it can be to cook and eat *en famille* when you're trying to lose weight, so these recipes are suitable for family eating but will work just as well if you are eating *à deux*, or even alone! You can always add extras such as pasta and potatoes for hungry partners and children.

If family eating isn't a concern, but running your hectic social life is, there's no need to worry. Whether cooking Sinner Dinners or Thinner Dinners, the recipes work equally well when entertaining. Your friends will love them as much as you do.

Thinner dinners

I am using the phrase Thinner Dinners lightly here – it's not diet food, it's good food! It's just a little lighter on the calories. You'll notice that there are more Thinner Dinners than Sinner Dinners. That's because you need to be more of a saint than a sinner when it comes to losing weight.

Vegetable Chilli

SERVES **6**   CALS: **213** per serving

I love spicy food. If you like the sound of this recipe, but aren't sure you can cope with the heat, it tastes just as good without the chilli. Just call it Vegetable Casserole instead.

2 tbsp olive oil
1 onion, sliced
2 red peppers, deseeded and cut into chunks
1 large carrot, peeled and cut into chunks
2 sweet potatoes, peeled and cut into chunks
1 butternut squash, peeled and cut into chunks
1 clove garlic, crushed
2 tsp chilli powder
400g can tomatoes
200ml vegetable stock
2 large courgettes, cut into chunks
400g can chickpeas or red kidney beans, drained and rinsed
1 tbsp yoghurt
½ a red and ½ a green chilli, deseeded and finely chopped
1 handful of spring onions, finely sliced
1 handful of fresh coriander leaves

Heat the oil in a pan over a medium heat and fry the onion for 5–8 minutes until soft. Add the peppers, carrot, sweet potatoes, butternut squash, garlic and chilli powder. Stir, then add the tomatoes and stock. Simmer for 20 minutes.

Add the courgettes and chickpeas, and simmer for 5–10 minutes until all the vegetables are tender. Transfer to a large serving dish, swirl the yoghurt on top, then sprinkle with fresh chillies, spring onions and coriander, and serve.

Warm Roasted Vegetable Salad

SERVES **4**   CALS: **217** per serving

This is one of my all-time favourites for a midweek supper. After a long day at work, I walk through the front door, chop up the veggies, put them in the oven, start on the homework (not mine, the children's) and by the time the homework's done, dinner is ready. If you don't have any 'homework' to do, you can luxuriate in the bath while this is cooking, or even better, go for a walk or jog around the block.

1 large red onion
1 aubergine
1 red pepper, deseeded
1 orange pepper, deseeded
1 large courgette
4 large tomatoes, halved
3 garlic cloves, cut into thin slices
1–4 tbsp olive oil
2 tbsp extra virgin olive oil
1 tbsp balsamic vinegar
1 tbsp fresh basil leaves
4 tbsp freshly grated Parmesan cheese
sea salt and freshly ground black pepper

Preheat the oven to 200°C/Gas 6. Cut the onion, aubergine, peppers and courgette into even-sized wedges. Put in a roasting tin, add the tomatoes and scatter over the garlic. Pour over 2 tbsp of the olive oil and mix well to ensure all the vegetables are coated. Season with salt and pepper. Roast for 40 minutes or until tender. Add a little extra oil if it gets too dry.

Meanwhile, put the vinegar and 1 tbsp extra virgin olive oil in a screwtop jar and season lightly with salt and pepper. Shake until blended.

Arrange the roasted vegetables on a serving dish and pour over the dressing. Sprinkle over the basil and Parmesan, and serve warm.

· ·

Jane Tip » *This is a very light supper. Great if you've had one of those weeks when sticking to your calorie allowance has been tough. If you wish to add extras, either for yourself or the family while the veggies are roasting, put a chicken breast in the oven for each person. Brush it with red pesto, add a basil leaf and wrap it in foil to keep it moist – and hey presto, it's done.*

Check the label for the size of your chicken breasts: on average they weigh around 125g and will add an extra 170 calories to this recipe. A teaspoon of shop-bought red pesto will add a further 50 calories.

· ·

Olivia's Ratatouille

SERVES 2   CALS: 200 per serving

My 16-year-old daughter Olivia is a very prolific cook. I often arrive home to find her following quite complex recipes and producing delicious dishes. This ratatouille is her very own recipe. It's quick and easy and makes a great Thinner Dinner, as it's so low in calories. I often make it on a Monday night, particularly if I've over-indulged at the weekend. The whole family love it and it can easily be made more substantial if necessary.

>   2 tbsp olive oil
>   1 red onion, finely sliced
>   2 x 400g cans chopped tomatoes
>   2 garlic cloves, finely sliced
>   2 red peppers, cut into chunks
>   2 aubergines, cut into rings
>   3 courgettes, cut into strips
>   a handful of fresh herb leaves, chopped, to serve

Heat ½ tbsp of the oil in a large pan over a medium heat and cook the onion and garlic for 5–8 minutes until they are golden and soft. Add the tomatoes and bring to the boil, then simmer for 5 minutes, or until slightly reduced. Remove from the heat.

Heat a ridged griddle. Put the peppers in a large bowl and drizzle over ½ tbsp olive oil, then toss them to cover with oil and transfer to the hot griddle. Cook, turning occasionally, so that they cook on both sides. Add to the tomato sauce. Cook the aubergines and courgettes in the same way and add to the tomatoes in the pan. Stir to make sure they are well combined, then gently reheat. Season to taste. Add the herb leaves, then serve.

Jane Tip ≫ *Olivia likes to serve this with chickpeas – allow ½ can per person and 145 calories. It goes equally well with pasta, rice, crusty bread, grated cheese, mozzarella, feta cheese, grilled chicken or fish – the list goes on and on. Check out the calorie chart on pages 262–70, so that you can be 100 per cent sure about exactly how many calories you're adding. For me, it's the ultimate Thinner Dinner, if you have had an indulgent weekend, and it needs nothing extra.*

Bear in mind that unless you add in extras, this dish contains no protein. So make sure you get your protein fix at some other time in the day.

Salmon Fillet with Roasted Cherry Tomatoes and Lemon

SERVES 4 **CALS: 373** per serving

A rainbow on a plate – this salmon dish looks and tastes bright, fresh and clean. I love serving it with a punchy-tasting watercress salad, but it works equally well with rocket, radish and sorrel.

12–18 cherry tomatoes
1 tbsp olive oil, plus extra for drizzling
4 salmon fillets, about 175g each
2 bunches of asparagus spears
1 tbsp chopped fresh dill leaves
zest and juice of 1 lemon
freshly ground black pepper
1 bunch of watercress, to serve

Preheat the oven to 190°C/Gas 5. Put the cherry tomatoes in a small baking dish, drizzle with olive oil and roast for 15–20 minutes until softened. Put the salmon fillets in a roasting tin and drizzle with olive oil and lemon juice. Season with pepper. Cook in the oven for 10–12 minutes.

Meanwhile, snap off any woody ends from the asparagus stalks at the point where they break easily and discard. Cook the asparagus for 2–3 minutes in boiling water – no more. Drain in a colander and rinse immediately under cold water, then put to one side.

Add the dill and lemon zest to the softly roasted tomatoes and mix thoroughly to make a dressing-like consistency. Divide the asparagus and salmon among 4 plates, then spoon the tomato mixture over each one. Season with salt and pepper and serve with a watercress salad.

....

Jane Tip ≫ *I rarely add anything to this salmon fillet recipe, but steamed new potatoes in summer or a jacket potato in winter would work well. The new potatoes will be an extra 75 cals for 100g – I wish I could tell you how many new potatoes that would be, but they vary so much in size, so on this occasion you will have to weigh them! A medium-size jacket potato will add around 250 cals.*

A diet rich in omega-3 fatty acids, found in salmon and other oily fish, helps cut your risk of heart disease.

....

Monkfish and Asparagus Stir-fry with Lime

SERVES **4**   CALS: **199** per serving

Quick, light and healthy, this recipe has a lovely combination of flavours. I especially love the zingy, tingly freshness of the lime.

500g monkfish fillet
150g asparagus
4 tbsp sunflower oil
2 courgettes, halved lengthways and sliced
1 red pepper, deseeded and sliced
2 garlic cloves, finely chopped
100g mangetouts
1 tbsp freshly grated lemongrass stalk
2.5cm fresh root ginger, peeled and grated
juice of 1–2 limes, to taste
fresh coriander leaves, finely chopped
sea salt and freshly ground black pepper

Remove the membrane from the fish and cut into thin slices (or ask your fishmonger to do this). Cover with clingfilm and leave to one side. Snap off any woody ends from the asparagus stalks at the point where they break easily and discard. Leave to one side.

Heat 2 tbsp of the oil in a wok or large frying pan over a medium heat. Add the courgettes and stir-fry for 2 minutes. Add the red pepper and garlic, and cook for a further 2 minutes, add the asparagus and cook for 1 minute, then add the mangetouts and cook for 2 minutes. Transfer the vegetables to a plate.

Heat the remaining oil in the wok and stir-fry the fish for 5 minutes, or until cooked through. Transfer the fish to another plate. Finally, put the lemongrass and ginger in the wok. Add the fish and half the lime juice, then stir-fry over a medium heat for a few seconds. Add the vegetables and stir-fry for 1 minute. Season, then taste and add more lime if needed. Sprinkle with coriander, then serve.

••

Jane Tip » *I eat this with lots of freshly steamed green beans and a dash of soy sauce. If you have enough calories in the bank to add noodles, allow 227 calories for a 125g serving. If you want the substance but not the calories, simply halve your noodle serving.*

Limes are rich in vitamin C – great for boosting the immune system.

••

Chilli Tuna Steak

SERVES 4 **CALS: 421** per serving

I love this recipe on a warm summer evening, eating around the barbecue – and it makes a healthy change from sausages and burgers. But don't just use this recipe in summer – it works just as well in a ridged griddle pan in midwinter. The heat from the chilli will soon warm you up.

This is what I call a 'make-it-the-night-before' recipe. Sounds too much like hard work? Actually, it can make your life easier. Simply set a reminder on your phone, get home, get going and then relax. Tomorrow's dinner is already sorted! (The tuna is marinated overnight; you can marinate it on the same day, but do try to leave at least 1 hour of marinating time. The longer you marinate, the more intense the flavour.)

4 tbsp olive oil
1½ tbsp lime juice
2 garlic cloves, crushed
1 small red chilli, deseeded and finely chopped
3 tbsp chopped fresh herb leaves
4 tuna steaks (maximum 150g each)
100g watercress
sea salt and freshly ground black pepper

Start preparations the evening before. Put the oil in a bowl and add 2 tbsp water, then whisk until thick and creamy. Continue to whisk, adding the lime juice, garlic, chilli and herbs to make a marinade. Season with salt and pepper. Put the tuna in a shallow ceramic dish and pour over over two-thirds of the marinade (put the remaining marinade in a small jug or bowl). Cover and leave to chill overnight.

When you're ready to cook, heat the barbecue or ridged griddle pan until smoking hot, then before you cook, turn it down to medium. Grill or griddle the tuna for about 2 minutes on either side until cooked on the outside but still rare in the centre. Put a large handful of watercress on each of 4 serving plates and put the tuna steak on top. Drizzle over the remaining marinade and serve.

· ·

Jane Tip ≫ *Serve with roasted tomatoes – they are rich in lycopene, an antioxidant that helps protect the body against a host of conditions.*

· ·

Plaice with Tomato Tapenade

SERVES **4**   CALS: **410** per serving

Ready in minutes, this is a good, easy midweek supper. I've used plaice, but it works equally well with most fish. The gutsy tomato tapenade is bursting with flavour. I love it!

    4 large ripe tomatoes
    1 tbsp black olives
    1 tbsp olive oil
    2 garlic cloves, peeled and left whole
    180g sun-dried tomatoes in olive oil, drained
    4 plaice fillets, about 180g each
    1 handful of fresh basil leaves
    sea salt and freshly ground black pepper

Preheat the oven to 190°C/Gas 5. Put the fresh tomatoes, olives, oil, garlic and sun-dried tomatoes into a food processor and blitz, or use a sharp knife to chop everything finely; this will give you a different texture, but the same taste sensation. Add salt and pepper to taste.

Spoon this tapenade mixture onto the plaice fillets. Put the plaice onto a baking tray and bake for 15 minutes or until the fish is cooked through. Remove from the oven and sprinkle a handful of basil over the top before serving.

· ·

Jane Tip » *I enjoy this dish with mangetouts and green beans but if you want to add potatoes, simple jacket potatoes with a sprinkling of cheese work well, but do make sure you have enough calories in the bank for this luxury. Allow a budget of 197 for your potato and another 123 calories for just 30g of grated Cheddar cheese.*

· ·

Salmon with Chilli, Ginger and Courgettes

SERVES 4   CALS: 437 per serving

Here is a lovely, fresh-tasting dish, with a simply gorgeous combination of Asian flavours. The recipe may appear complicated, but it is in fact incredibly simple to follow. That said, I usually make it at the weekend, because although it's simple, there is slightly more fiddling around compared with many of my Thinner Dinners – but trust me, even with the fiddling around, it's so worth it!

250ml mirin
200g pak choi
4 fish fillets, such as salmon (about 150–175g each)
4 garlic cloves, finely sliced
100ml soy sauce
3 red chillies, deseeded and finely chopped
8 spring onions, finely shredded
1.5cm fresh root ginger, peeled and grated
2 tbsp olive oil
8 courgettes, cut into 2cm-wide strips lengthways
1 handful of fresh coriander leaves, chopped
2 limes, cut into wedges, to serve

Put 200ml of the mirin in a pan over a medium-high heat and bring it to the boil, then simmer until reduced by half. Leave to cool.

Meanwhile, preheat the oven to 180°C/Gas 4. Cut a large rectangle of foil, big enough to make a large envelope to hold all the fish fillets. Put the pak choi on the foil, followed by the fish, then half the garlic, 50ml of the soy sauce, the remaining 50ml of the mirin and 1 chopped chilli, then season to taste. Put the fish parcels in the oven and cook for 20 minutes.

Add the remaining soy sauce to the pan with the reduced, cooled mirin and add 4 of the spring onions, the remaining garlic cloves and chillies and the ginger. Stir to make a sauce.

Heat the oil in a large frying pan until hot. Score the white, fleshy side of the courgettes in a criss-cross pattern. Lower the courgettes into the pan and lightly fry on both sides until the flesh is golden. Once cooked, dab off the excess oil on kitchen paper and put onto a baking tray, skin-side down. Carefully spoon the sauce over, dividing it as you go between each courgette. Cook in the oven for 5–10 minutes until tender.

Open the parcel to check that the fish is cooked through, and give it a few more minutes if necessary. Transfer the fish to a serving dish. Scatter over the remaining spring onions and all the coriander. Remove the courgettes from the oven, and arrange them around the fish, pouring the remaining sauce from the baking tray over them. Serve with the lime wedges.

Jane Tip » *When I tested this recipe I tried it out on my teenagers. I thought they'd ask for noodles to accompany the salmon and courgettes, but they all loved it just as it is. So, guided by them, I suggest you enjoy this one 'noodle free'.*

Fluffy Prawn Omelette

SERVES **2** CALS: **200** per serving

When you are completely exhausted and thinking of turning to the toaster for a quick and easy super, think again! This omelette hits the spot. I love to cook this when I'm home alone – all you have to do is halve the ingredients. It couldn't be simpler, and you have dinner for one in a matter of minutes. It's so much better than that toast and Marmite!

> 115g cooked, peeled prawns
> 4 spring onions, finely chopped
> 1 small courgette, finely chopped
> 4 medium free-range eggs, separated
> a few dashes of Tabasco, to taste
> 3 tbsp milk
> 1 tbsp olive oil
> 25g Cheddar cheese, grated
> freshly ground black pepper

Mix the prawns, spring onions and courgettes in a bowl and leave to one side. Put the egg yolks in a bowl and beat with the Tabasco, milk and pepper to taste. Leave to one side. In a separate bowl, whisk the egg whites until stiff, then fold in the yolk mixture.

Heat the oil in a large frying pan and pour in the egg mixture. Cook for 4–6 minutes until lightly set. Preheat the grill. Spoon the prawn mixture on top of the eggs and sprinkle with cheese. Grill for 2–3 minutes. Cut into wedges and serve.

···

Jane Tip » *Adding a crunchy, munchy green salad doesn't take much effort and will contribute towards your five-a-day.*

···

Chicken Laksa

SERVES **4**   CALS: **317** per serving

This was the first ever recipe I created for a client. It's now become an all-time Jane Plan favourite. Warming, soothing and utterly delicious – it's love in a bowl.

1 tsp sunflower oil
2 shallots, finely chopped
2 red chillies, deseeded and chopped
5cm piece of fresh root ginger, peeled and finely sliced
2 lemongrass stalks, outer leaves removed, finely chopped
400g chicken breasts, sliced
600ml chicken stock
2 tbsp fish sauce
1 tbsp soft brown sugar or palm sugar
a few large handfuls of baby leaf spinach
200ml low-fat coconut milk
juice of 2 limes
2 bundles of thin rice noodles
fresh coriander leaves and lime wedges, to serve

Heat the oil in a pan over a medium heat and cook the shallots, chillies and ginger for 2 minutes. Add the lemongrass, chicken and stock, and bring to a simmer. Stir in the fish sauce and sugar, and simmer for 10 minutes or until the chicken is cooked. Add the baby spinach, coconut milk and lime juice, then simmer until the spinach wilts.

Cook the rice noodles according to the pack instructions and stir into the laksa. Divide among four bowls and garnish with fresh coriander and lime wedges, then serve.

Mediterranean Chicken with Pecorino Crust

SERVES **4**   CALS: **389** per serving

I usually make this at the weekend, because it takes a little more prep time than some of my other recipes. It's a Mediterranean classic, and it works well with Parmesan too!

400g aubergines, cut lengthways into thick slices
3 tbsp olive oil, plus extra for brushing
4 skinless chicken breasts, about 100g each
1 large red onion, finely sliced
400g can chopped tomatoes
3 garlic cloves, finely sliced
1 tsp dried oregano
1 tbsp chopped fresh basil leaves
1 handful of pitted black olives
125g mozzarella, sliced
40g grated pecorino cheese
sea salt and freshly ground black pepper
green salad with fennel, to serve

Preheat the oven to 180°C/Gas 4 and preheat the grill. Put the aubergine slices on a baking sheet. Brush with a little oil and cook under the grill until each side is lightly browned.

Meanwhile, heat 2 tbsp of the olive oil in a frying pan over a medium heat and gently fry the chicken breasts until slightly coloured. Remove from the pan from the heat and add the remaining oil, then fry the onion for 5–8 minutes until softened. Add the tomatoes and garlic, and season to taste, then stir in the oregano and add the basil leaves and olives.

Spoon the tomato and olive mixture into an ovenproof dish. Put the chicken on top and cover the chicken with the aubergine and mozzarella. Sprinkle over the grated pecorino, then cook for 25–35 minutes. Serve with a salad of mixed green leaves and sliced fennel.

Jane Tip ≫ *The fennel added to the salad to serve works well with the tomatoey flavours.*

Chilli Lime Chicken with a Yoghurt Dipping Sauce

SERVES 4   CALS: **200** per serving

This is a 'do-it-the-night-before' recipe – it takes just a tiny amount of planning to make a massively delicious meal that's big on taste but low in calories. There's a fair amount of chilli in the marinade, so if you prefer a cooler mix, reduce the amount. This recipe is great for serving solo – as it's incredibly easy to reduce the ingredients to make it suitable for one.

3 tbsp chilli powder
2 tbsp extra virgin olive oil
2 tsp lime zest
3 tbsp lime juice
3 garlic cloves, crushed
1 tsp ground coriander
1 tsp ground cumin
1 tsp cayenne pepper
a pinch of ground cinnamon
4 skinless chicken breasts, about 100g each
sea salt and freshly ground black pepper
steamed vegetables, to serve

For the yoghurt dipping sauce
400g low-fat yoghurt
½ cucumber, diced
3 spring onions, sliced
1 handful of fresh mint leaves, finely chopped

Start preparations the evening before. Combine the chilli powder and oil in a small bowl with the lime zest and juice, garlic, coriander, cumin, cayenne pepper, cinnamon, and salt and pepper, to form a wet paste. Generously smear this spice rub all over the chicken then cover and chill overnight.

When you get home from work the following day, heat the oven to 200°C/Gas 6 and put the chicken into a roasting tin. Cook in the oven for 30 minutes or until the chicken is cooked through. (Alternatively, cook in a griddle pan.)

To make the dipping sauce, mix the yoghurt with the cucumber, spring onions and mint. Serve with the chicken and steamed vegetables (see tip).

••

Jane Tip » *I like to prepare a platter of steamed vegetables to go with this dish: Chantenay carrots, mangetouts and leeks work well. I give them a quick spritz of freshly squeezed lime juice, then put the cooked chicken on top. I then drizzle the yoghurt mixture over the top of the chicken, leaving some in the bowl to put on the table, so that everyone can serve themselves. If I'm super-stressed and far too busy to think, I buy tzatziki instead, which saves making the yoghurt sauce.*

Aduki beans add extra bulk here. I tend to use canned beans for convenience. Warm them gently in a pan, add a squeeze of lemon and leave in the middle of the table for everyone to help themselves. A tablespoon of aduki beans (30g) is about 37 calories.

••

Chicken tray bakes

There's nothing like a chicken tray bake. I make them all the time and usually throw in whatever veggies I have to hand, so feel free to ad-lib here. The great thing about a tray bake is that there is hardly any preparation, and virtually no washing up. And you get a meal ready in just a few minutes that tastes delicious. I love using these recipes on a busy week-day night. I pop everything into the baking tray, whiz upstairs to change out of my work clothes, then settle down to chat to the children and help with the homework. By the time all that's done, dinner is ready. If you are lucky enough not to have to supervise homework, then why not relax in a long hot bath, while dinner literally 'makes itself'.

I was going to think up some exotic names for them, but ultimately they are simply Chicken Tray Bakes, and because Jane Plan is all about simplicity, I decided to retain the names we use – The Mediterranean One, The Root Vegetable One and The Filling One.

You will probably notice that all the chicken tray bakes suggest one chicken thigh per person with the skin on. Of course, that means it's higher in fat, but somehow roasted chicken thigh just doesn't taste the same without the skin, and as chicken thighs are relatively small, they make great portion-controlled meals. If you do want to boost the calories, you could add an extra thigh at 130 calories, or use a chicken leg at 230 calories. Personally, I like the perfectly portioned thigh. Sometimes I pop a bowl of minted yoghurt with spring onions stirred in to it, on the table. It tastes great as a side dipping sauce.

If you like the idea of a tray bake but don't eat meat, you can roast any combination of vegetables and add a sprinkle of feta cheese. The great thing about feta is that it works equally well with all three of the tray bakes here, as its strong flavour is not diluted by the powerful flavours of the roasted vegetables.

The Mediterranean One

SERVES **4**   CALS: **268** per serving

1 red onion, cut into wedges
2 red peppers, deseeded and cut into chunks
2 courgettes, cut into chunks
1 small aubergine, cut into chunks
4 tomatoes, halved, or 8 small vine tomatoes left whole
4 tbsp olive oil, plus extra for drizzling
4 chicken thighs, with skin
1 tbsp pitted black olives
1 handful of fresh basil leaves, chopped
sea salt and freshly ground black pepper
mixed salad of endive, radicchio, green leaves and herbs,
    to serve

Preheat the oven to 200°C/Gas 6. Put all the vegetables and the tomatoes in a shallow roasting tin. Pour over the olive oil and give everything a good mix until well coated (your hands are easiest for this).

Put the chicken, skin-side up, on top of the vegetables. Season everything with salt and pepper and drizzle a little oil over the chicken. Roast for 20 minutes, then scatter the black olives on top and return the tin to the oven for another 15 minutes or until the vegetables are soft and the chicken is golden and the juices run clear when the flesh is pierced with a sharp knife. Scatter the basil over the top before serving. Serve with a mixed salad.

The Root Vegetable One

SERVES 4 CALS: 324 per serving

You can add extra feta cheese if you like – allow another 50 calories for every extra 20g of feta per person.

- 2 beetroots, peeled and cut into discs
- 1 red onion, cut into wedges
- 1 small butternut squash, peeled and cut into discs
- 2 large carrots, cut lengthways into thick wedges
- 4 tbsp olive oil, plus extra for drizzling
- 4 chicken thighs, with skin
- 1 handful of fresh sage leaves, finely chopped
- 80g feta cheese, crumbled
- sea salt and freshly ground black pepper

Preheat the oven to 200°C/Gas 6. Put the beetroots in a roasting tin and toss with a little of the oil. Cook in the oven for 10 minutes.

Add all the remaining vegetables to the tin and pour over the remaining oil, then give everything a good mix until well coated (your hands are easiest for this).

Put the chicken, skin-side up, on top of the vegetables. Season everything with salt and pepper and drizzle a little oil over the chicken. Roast for 20 minutes, then scatter the sage leaves on top and return to the oven for another 15 minutes or until the vegetables are soft and the chicken is golden and the juices run clear when the flesh is pierced with a sharp knife. Scatter over the feta cheese before serving.

The Filling One

SERVES **4**   CALS: **299** per serving

This tray bake has lots of lovely Mediterranean veggies, but also potatoes, which makes it tasty and filling.

- 1 red onion, cut into wedges
- 4 medium potatoes, unpeeled and cut into small cubes
- 1 courgette, cut into chunks
- 1 aubergine, cut into chunks
- 1 fennel bulb, cut into slices
- 4 garlic cloves, unpeeled
- 4 tbsp olive oil
- 4 chicken thighs, with skin
- a sprinkle of dried rosemary
- a small handful of fresh basil leaves
- sea salt and freshly ground black pepper

Preheat the oven to 200°C/Gas 6. Put all the vegetables and the garlic in a shallow roasting tin. Put the chicken, skin-side up, on top of the vegetables. Season everything with salt and pepper and scatter the rosemary over the top. Pour over the olive oil and mix everything together until well coated (your hands are easiest for this).

Roast for 35 minutes or until the vegetables are soft and the chicken is golden and the juices run clear when the flesh is pierced with a sharp knife. Scatter the basil over the top before serving.

....

Jane Tip ≫ *This is equally gorgeous with cod steak or even salmon – start roasting the vegetables, then add the fish after the first 15 minutes, as the fish will cook faster than the chicken.*

....

Griddled Chicken with Quinoa

SERVES **4**   CALS: **366** per serving

Quinoa is a complete protein and has been recognised by the United Nations as a super-crop for its health benefits.

225g quinoa
1½ tbsp extra virgin olive oil
1 red chilli, deseeded and finely chopped
½ tsp dried oregano
1 garlic clove, crushed
400g chicken mini-fillets
300g vine tomatoes, roughly chopped
1 handful of pitted black Kalamata olives
1 red onion, finely sliced
1 small bunch of mint leaves, chopped
zest and juice of ½ lemon
sea salt and freshly ground black pepper
rocket salad, to serve

Cook the quinoa according to the pack instructions, then rinse in cold water and drain thoroughly in a colander.

Meanwhile, put 1 tbsp of the olive oil in a dish large enough to hold the chicken in one layer and stir in the chilli, oregano and garlic. Add the chicken fillets and coat with the oil mixture. Leave to marinate for a minimum of 10 minutes. Heat a ridged griddle pan. Put the chicken in the griddle and cook for 3–4 minutes on each side until cooked through. Transfer to a plate, and leave to one side.

Put the tomatoes, olives, onion and mint into a bowl. Toss in the cooked quinoa. Stir in the remaining olive oil and the lemon zest and juice. Season well. Serve the quinoa with the chicken fillets on top, and a simple rocket salad by the side.

Tandoori Lamb

SERVES **4** CALS: **281** per serving

Are you missing your Friday night takeaway? This healthy take on a classic Indian dish will make your mouth water – and it's a fraction of the calories of a typical takeaway.

juice of 1 lemon
2 tsp paprika
1 red onion, finely chopped
400g lean stewing lamb, cut into cubes
sunflower oil, for brushing
iceberg lettuce salad, to serve

For the marinade
150ml low-fat Greek yogurt
1.5cm piece of fresh root ginger, peeled and grated
2 garlic cloves, crushed
⅓ tsp each of garam masala, ground cumin, chilli powder
   and turmeric

If possible, start preparations the night before. Put the lemon juice in a large shallow dish and add the paprika and red onion. Mix together well. Add the lamb to the dish and mix to ensure it is well covered by the juices. Leave to one side for 10 minutes.

Mix all the marinade ingredients together in a small bowl and pour over the lamb mixture. Give everything a good stir, then cover and chill for at least 1 hour or overnight.

Preheat the grill. Put the lamb in a roasting tin. Brush over a little oil and grill for 8 minutes on each side or until lightly charred and completely cooked through. Serve with a green salad.

Lemony Lamb with Rosemary, Mint and Broad Beans

SERVES 2   CALS: **300** per serving

This is a wonderful alternative to a classic roast lamb Sunday lunch. Forget about gravy and roast potatoes, instead savour the freshness of the flavours in this contemporary lamb dish. It works equally well for dinner too, and if you're cooking for friends and family you can simply double the ingredients.

Lamb is a rich source of protein and vitamins A, B_3, B_6 and B_{12} and it also contains healthy omega-3 fats. Griddling the meat will allow some of the fat to drain off during the cooking process.

150g low-fat natural yoghurt
2 tsp balsamic vinegar
juice of 1 lemon
1 tbsp chopped fresh mint leaves
1 tbsp chopped fresh rosemary leaves
180g lean lamb, cut into 3cm cubes
2 courgettes, diced
1 red pepper, cut into cubes
1 small red onion, cut into small wedges
200g frozen broad beans
1 tsp olive oil
sea salt and freshly ground black pepper

Put the yoghurt in a large bowl and add the balsamic vinegar, half the lemon juice, the mint and rosemary. Season with salt and pepper and mix together well. Add the lamb and mix well to ensure that each piece is coated. Leave to marinate for 10 minutes.

Heat a ridged griddle pan. Thread the lamb onto four metal skewers, alternating each cube with a piece of courgette, pepper and onion. Cook the lamb for 3–4 minutes, turning the skewers to ensure that each side is coloured. Meanwhile, put the broad beans in a steamer and steam over a high heat for 10 minutes or until just tender. Drizzle the warm broad beans with the olive oil and the remaining lemon juice. Put the broad beans on a platter and lay the lamb skewers on top, then serve.

••

Jane Tip » *Thinking of adding minted new potatoes? Allow 75 calories for 100g.*

••

Aubergine Curry

SERVES **4**   CALS: **243** per serving

- 1 tbsp coriander seeds
- ½ tbsp fennel seeds
- 6 cloves
- 2 star anise
- 2 tbsp sunflower oil
- ½ tsp ground turmeric
- 1 tsp sea salt
- 400ml coconut milk
- 2 tsp tamarind paste
- a small handful of fresh curry or coriander leaves
- 12 tomatoes (skinned and cored is best, but I frequently leave them just as they are, see tip)
- 1 large aubergine, cut into thumb-sized chunks
- 6 fresh mint leaves, chopped

Put the coriander seeds, fennel seeds, cloves and star anise in a small dry pan and lightly toast over a medium heat until the aromas are released. Remove from the heat. Heat the oil in a wide pan over a medium heat and add the toasted spices. Fry for 2 minutes, then add the turmeric and salt.

Pour in the coconut milk and stir in the tamarind paste and curry leaves. Bring to the boil and simmer gently for 15 minutes. Blend the mixture with a blender or food processor for 30 seconds, then remove from the heat and leave to infuse.

Pass the coconut sauce through a fine sieve and return it to the pan. Put the tomatoes and aubergine chunks into the sauce, then bring to the boil, reduce the heat and simmer for 15–20 minutes until softened and the sauce has reduced slightly. Taste and adjust the seasoning, then stir in the mint leaves and serve.

Jane Tip » *To peel tomatoes, plunge the tomatoes into boiling water for 30 seconds, then refresh in cold water. Peel away the skins, then halve and cut out the cores.*

Autumn is the time for aubergines. Make sure the flesh is white rather than green, which means the fruit is ripe. If there are lots of seeds it can mean the aubergines are over-ripe, but still perfectly usable; however, the flesh may be tougher and may soak up more oil while cooking. Calorie counters, beware!

Beef and Broccoli Stir-fry

SERVES 2 **CALS: 206** per serving

This is a fabulously fast Thinner Dinner, great after a long, hard day and packed with protein. I have used broccoli, mangetouts and peppers here, which provide a beautiful array of colours, but you can add any vegetables you fancy, and it will still taste delicious. Try carrot batons, pak choi, bean sprouts and shredded cabbage. With this dish, the world is your oyster.

2 tbsp soy sauce
3 tbsp sherry
1 tsp sugar
2 tbsp sunflower oil
1 red onion, thinly sliced
300g beef rump steak, cut into thin strips
300g broccoli florets
1 red pepper, deseeded and cut into strips
80g mangetouts
lime juice and chopped fresh coriander leaves,
   to serve (optional)

Put the soy sauce in a small bowl and add the sherry, sugar and 2 tbsp water. Mix well, then leave to one side. Heat the oil in a large frying pan or wok, add the onion and beef, and stir-fry quickly until the beef is lightly browned. Transfer to a plate.

Add the broccoli to the pan and stir-fry for 1 minute, then add the pepper and mangetouts. Add the soy mixture. Bring to the boil, then cover and simmer for 3–5 minutes until the broccoli is just tender.

Tip the beef and onion back into the pan and heat through briefly before serving. It's delicious with a squeeze of lime and fresh coriander, if you like.

••

Jane Tip ≫ *If you want to add rice, cook 75g raw rice per person and take 265 calories out of your calorie savings account.*

••

Mediterranean Vegetables with Beef

SERVES **4**   CALS: **184** per serving

Adding anchovies to beef really brings out the flavour. This one-pot meal is deliciously soothing and bursting with flavour, and for a beef-based casserole it is surprisingly low in calories.

Stick to the quantities of beef I have suggested here, and you can enjoy a heart-warming, satisfying and comforting dish, without the calories usually associated with this type of eating.

> 1 tbsp olive oil
> 250g lean beef fillet, trimmed of any fat and thinly sliced
> 140g shallots, halved
> 2 large courgettes, cut into chunks
> 1 red, 1 orange and 1 green pepper, deseeded and cut into chunks
> 1 garlic clove, sliced
> 4 anchovy fillets, cut into tiny pieces
> 150ml vegetable stock
> 250g cherry tomatoes
> 2 tsp fresh rosemary leaves
> sea salt and freshly ground black pepper

Heat the oil in a large, heavy-based frying pan over a high heat. Cook the beef and shallots for 2–3 minutes until golden. Add the courgettes and stir-fry for 3–4 minutes until beginning to soften.

Add the peppers, garlic and anchovies. Reduce the heat to medium and cook for 4–5 minutes until they start to soften. Pour in the stock and stir to coat. Add the tomatoes and season with salt and pepper, then cover with a lid and simmer, stirring occasionally, until the vegetables are tender and the meat is cooked through. Taste and adjust the seasoning if needed.

Stir in the rosemary and serve.

....

Jane Tip » *If you want to add mashed potatoes, they will soak up all the delicious juices. But remember: a tennis ball-size serving of mashed potato is about 162 calories.*

For a deeper, more intense flavour, you can add more anchovies. They are also a great source of calcium.

....

Courgette Spaghetti

People who are trying to lose weight often tell me that although they keep away from pasta they really miss it. Using courgette spaghetti, rather than your usual pasta, will help you overcome this pasta craving, and it works well with all pasta sauces. What's more, courgettes are a good source of vitamin C.

CALS: **93** (3 large courgettes per person)

Cut the courgettes into thin slices lengthways, and then cut each slice into thin strips to create spaghetti-like strips. If you are not skilled with the knife, you can find kitchen gadgets – such as a mandoline – to help you make them into spaghetti-like strips.

Boil the courgette strips in water for 2 minutes, drain and serve with your favourite spaghetti sauce, such as the Prawn Pasta that follows.

Prawn Pasta

SERVES **4**   CALS: **202** for the sauce

This can be served with your usual pasta or the courgette spaghetti on the previous page. As I like to save on calories, I would go for the courgette spaghetti every time, but as long as you stay within your calorie allowance, you can enjoy either.

3 tbsp olive oil
1 large shallot, chopped
1 garlic clove, finely sliced
1 handful of chopped fresh parsley leaves, plus extra to serve
½ tsp dried chilli flakes
400g can chopped tomatoes
250ml dry white wine
450g peeled prawns, thawed if frozen
sea salt and freshly ground black pepper
courgette spaghetti or pasta, to serve

Put the oil in a wide-based, shallow pan over a medium heat, add the shallot, and cook for 5 minutes or until it softens but not browns. Add the garlic, parsley and chilli flakes, stir for 1 minute then add the tomatoes. Pour in the wine then bring to the boil and simmer the sauce for 10 minutes. Add the prawns and cook for 3–5 minutes until they are heated through.

If you are serving the sauce with courgette spaghetti, add it to the pan of boiling water about 3 minutes before you are ready to serve. If using pasta, allow longer, depending on the type of pasta you are using, and cook it according to the pack instructions. Drain in a colander. Put the courgette spaghetti or pasta in a serving dish, add the sauce and stir well, mixing everything together. Serve with more parsley on top.

Jane Tip » *If you are having standard pasta, allow 75g per person and 265 calories extra.*

Cauliflower Rice

CALS: **50** for a 160g portion

At Jane Plan, one of the most frequently asked questions is 'What about rice?', 'What can I eat instead?' I stumbled across this recipe, and it seems to really hit the spot – and even better, it freezes well. Try coconut oil to cook the 'rice'. It tastes really good with the cauliflower and works particularly well if you are making an Asian dish.

    1 large cauliflower, cut into florets
    a drizzle of coconut oil or olive oil
    sea salt and freshly ground black pepper
    a dash of spice of your choice (optional)

Put a handful of florets in the bowl of your food processor and process to chop finely and evenly, so that it looks like grains of rice. Repeat with the remaining cauliflower. (Alternatively, you can use a hand grater, although it will be more time-consuming.)

Heat a small amount of oil in a non-stick pan over a medium-high heat, add the cauliflower rice and cook for 5–10 minutes. Season with salt, pepper and another complementary spice, if you like.

Jane Tip » *Uncooked cauliflower rice freezes really well. If cooking the cauliflower rice from frozen, remove from the freezer and leave it to thaw while you are cooking your main dish.*

Sinner dinners

I thought long and hard about calling these Sinner Dinners, as I don't like the idea of demonising any food. What's more, all these recipes are deliciously healthy; however, I do think it's good to be aware that even healthy food can be calorie high.

These recipes are beautifully balanced and certainly not packed with ingredients you should necessarily be eating less of, but they are higher in calories than the Thinner Dinners. Try not to think of these recipes as 'naughty' but more as great food that's good to eat but not all the time. Before indulging in a Sinner Dinner, the secret is to check your calorie bank account and make sure you have enough credit.

Spicy Green Papaya Salad

SERVES **2** CALS: **562** per serving

I created this for one of my very first clients, who is now one of my best friends. Gen lost 5 stone (31.7kg) with Jane Plan – quite an achievement – and three years on she hasn't regained the weight! She needed a recipe to celebrate Chinese New Year – so I came up with this. It's worth noting, she made it without the nuts. The papaya for this dish should be very firm and when cut the flesh should be white to light orange in colour.

- 1 small or ½ a large green papaya
- 1 or 2 tomatoes, cut into long, thin strips
- 3 spring onions, sliced into long matchstick strips
- 1 red chilli, finely chopped (deseeded if you prefer a milder salad), or to taste
- 100g bean sprouts
- 50g fresh basil leaves, roughly chopped if large

125g honey-roasted or plain roasted peanuts,
   or glazed cashew nuts
1 handful of fresh coriander leaves

For the dressing
½ tsp shrimp paste
2 tbsp olive oil
a squeeze of lime juice, or to taste
2 tbsp fish sauce, or to taste
honey, to taste

To make the dressing, put all the dressing ingredients in a small bowl and mix well; make sure the shrimp paste and honey dissolve fully.

Peel the papaya, then slice it in half and remove all the seeds. Using the largest grater you have, grate the papaya and put it in a large bowl. Add the tomatoes, spring onions, chilli, beansprouts and most of the basil. Add the dressing and toss together.

Add the nuts, then toss again. Taste the salad – if not sweet enough, add a little more honey; if not salty enough, add a little more fish sauce; if too sweet or salty, add more lime juice; if you prefer it spicier, add more chilli. To serve, scoop the salad into individual bowls or onto a serving platter. Sprinkle with the remaining basil leaves and the coriander.

· ·

Jane Tip » *Who would have thought that a simple papaya salad could be so high in calories! It's the nuts – if you decide to leave them out you will save a massive 176 calories, but remember the nuts are the protein element of the meal.*

· ·

Melanzane alla Parmigiana

SERVES 4–6 **CALS: 525** per serving, if serving 4;
365 per serving, if serving 6

This is a firm family favourite and makes a wonderful change from classic lasagne. Do leave time to prepare it, however, as it always seems to take longer than you think. Making it for 6 will turn it into a Thinner Dinner.

2 tbsp olive oil, plus extra for brushing
3 garlic cloves, crushed
leaves from 3 fresh thyme sprigs
4 x 400g cans chopped tomatoes
250ml red wine
¼ tsp dried oregano
6 large aubergines, very thinly sliced lengthways
2 x 125g mozzarella balls, sliced
100g finely grated Parmesan cheese
1 handful of fresh basil leaves
85g white breadcrumbs
sea salt and freshly ground black pepper
salad, to serve

Preheat the oven to 200°C/Gas 6. Heat the oil in a large frying pan or wide pan over a medium heat, add the garlic and thyme, and cook gently for 5 minutes. Add the tomatoes, wine and oregano, then bring to the boil and reduce the heat. Simmer for 20–25 minutes until slightly thickened.

Meanwhile, heat a ridged griddle pan or frying pan over a medium-high heat. Brush the aubergine slices on both sides with olive oil, then griddle in batches. Each slice should be softened and slightly charred; if necessary, reduce the heat so that the aubergines don't char before softening. Put the slices on a plate lined with kitchen paper and dab the slices with more paper to absorb the oil.

Spread a fifth of the tomato sauce over the base of a large baking dish. Top the sauce with a layer of half the aubergine slices, then season well. Spoon over a quarter of the remaining sauce, then scatter over half the mozzarella, a little Parmesan and some basil leaves. Repeat the layering up, finishing with the last of the tomato sauce. Mix together the breadcrumbs and remaining Parmesan and scatter it over the top. Cook in the oven for 20 minutes or until golden. Serve with salad.

· ·

Jane Tip » *I serve this for friends and family with a simple salad, although my son loves it with pesto beans on the side. To make pesto beans, steam green beans then tip into the pan. Add a drizzle of pesto sauce while they are still warm in the pan. Pour onto a serving plate and top with pine nuts. 160g of green beans is 38 calories, a teaspoon of pesto is 50 calories and a teaspoon of pine nuts is 68 calories. As you can see, it's often the added extras that make the difference when it comes to counting calories.*

· ·

Sea Bream with Mexican Salsa

SERVES 4 CALS: 582 per serving with sea bream (500g);
542 per serving with mackerel (200g)

This recipe needs no introduction – its deliciousness speaks for itself. Just look at the clean ingredients – they shout 'goodness' at the top of their voices. And there is nothing like being presented with a whole fish – it really is a fish-lover's treat. You can also make this with mackerel.

4 whole sea bream or mackerel, de-scaled and cleaned
   (ask your fishmonger to do this)
1 tbsp olive oil
2 tbsp Cajun seasoning
mixed salad, to serve

For the salsa
5 tomatoes, chopped
1 red chilli, deseeded and finely chopped
1 ripe avocado, halved, stoned, peeled and diced
2 spring onions, sliced
1 small bunch of fresh coriander, chopped
zest and juice of 1 lime
sea salt and freshly ground black pepper

Preheat the oven to 200°C/Gas 6 and line a baking tray with foil. Make 3–4 slashes on each side of the fish. Drizzle over the olive oil and sprinkle with the Cajun seasoning. Put the fish on the prepared baking tray and cook in the oven for 12–15 minutes until just cooked through.

Preheat the grill to high and cook the fish for 2–3 minutes to char the skin. Cover and leave to rest for a few minutes.

To make the salsa, put the tomatoes in a bowl and add the chilli, avocado, spring onions, coriander, lime juice and zest. Season and mix well. Serve the fish with the salsa and a simple mixed salad.

. . . .

Jane Tip ≫ *If you want to halve the calories, share your sea bream with another person.*

Fish is a good source of essential vitamins, such as niacin, and minerals, such as selenium and iodine; however, different types of fish have different health benefits. Mackerel is an oily fish, rich in omega-3 fatty acids, which help prevent heart disease. Bream is a white fish, which is very low in fat. It does contain omega-3 fatty acids, but at much lower levels than oily fish.

. . . .

Seafood Risotto

SERVES 2   CALS: 601 per serving

This is one of my family favourites – it always brings back memories of happy, sunny Mediterranean holidays. The recipe calls for fish stock; I use a stock cube here, but you can buy fish stock now from most supermarkets. The stock needs to be simmering, so heat it in a pan and ladle it out from the pan into the risotto as you cook it. You will also need cooked squid and prawns, but if you prefer, you can buy a bag of mixed cooked seafood (sometimes called seafood cocktail) and use 200g of this instead of the prawns and squid.

    2 tbsp olive oil
    2 banana shallots or 1 onion, chopped
    2 garlic cloves, crushed
    250ml dry white wine or vermouth
    150g Arborio rice
    500ml hot fish stock
    100g cooked squid
    100g cooked peeled prawns
    4 large tomatoes, finely chopped
    1 handful of fresh dill and parsley leaves
    sea salt and freshly ground black pepper
    lime juice, lime wedges and salad, to serve

Heat the oil in a pan and add the shallots and garlic. Cook for 5–8 minutes until softened, then add the wine and the rice. Stir to coat the rice in the oil.

Gradually add the simmering stock, a ladleful at a time, stirring continuously and ensuring that the rice has absorbed the stock before adding another ladleful. After about 20 minutes almost all the liquid will have been absorbed and the rice should be al dente (tender but with a bite in the centre).

Add the seafood, stirring it into the rice until it has heated through. Add the tomatoes and briefly stir again, making sure the seafood is warmed through, but don't overcook. Season to taste with salt and pepper. Serve sprinkled with dill and parsley, with a squeeze of lime juice, and have extra lime wedges and a salad on the side.

· ·

Jane Tip » *I like to add a simple mixed salad too – fennel, endive and rocket work well here.*

You can also serve this dish to four people rather than two, which instantly halves the calories, turning your Sinner Dinner into a Thinner Dinner. If you decide to do this, make sure you accompany it with a large salad.

· ·

One-pan Chicken and Chorizo Casserole

SERVES 4 CALS: 561 per serving

This is a simple and classic combination of flavours that produce a lovely rich smoky dish that everyone will love.

    200g chorizo, cut into 1cm slices
    2 garlic cloves, crushed
    1 red onion, sliced
    8 skinless chicken thighs
    150ml red wine
    400g can chopped tomatoes
    1 handful of fresh parsley leaves, chopped
    sea salt and freshly ground black pepper
    watercress salad, to serve

Preheat the oven to 180°C/Gas 4. Heat a flameproof casserole over a medium heat and fry the chorizo, garlic and onion for 5 minutes. Remove from the casserole and add the chicken. Brown the chicken until golden on both sides, then return the chorizo and onion to the casserole with the chicken. Pour over the wine and tomatoes.

Season with salt and pepper, cover and cook in the oven for 40 minutes or until the chicken is cooked through. Stir in the parsley and serve with a watercress salad.

· ·

Jane Tip » *I have not included potatoes, pasta or rice here, and the recipe already hits the 500-plus calorie mark. Before adding in any extras, do check your calorie allowance.*

· ·

Slow Roast Leg of Lamb

SERVES **6**   CALS: **682** per serving

This is slow cooking at its best. The aromas of the lamb as it is gently cooking are so seductive that I can never resist popping into the kitchen to take a peek.

1.8kg leg of lamb
8 garlic cloves, cut into slivers
1 handful of fresh rosemary leaves
6 anchovy fillets, cut into slivers
2 x 400g cans of butter beans, drained and rinsed
400g can chopped tomatoes
500ml red wine
150ml lamb stock (use a stock cube), plus extra if needed
2 leeks, cut into 5cm pieces
200g carrots, sliced lengthways into thick batons
steamed vegetables, to serve

Preheat the oven to 180°C/Gas 4. Make fine incisions in the lamb and insert slivers of four of the garlic cloves, and the rosemary and anchovies.

Put the beans in a casserole and add the tomatoes, then pour over the wine and stock. Stir in the remaining garlic, and add the leeks and carrots. Put the lamb on top, then cover and cook in the oven for 3–3½ hours until the lamb is tender, adding more stock if needed. Serve with steamed vegetables.

....

Jane Tip » *Steamed green beans, sugar snap peas and asparagus add colour, texture and a fresh, clean flavour and make a lovely side dish.*

....

Spring Lamb Moroccan-style

SERVES **4**   CALS: **719** per serving

This recipe is perfect when lamb is at its best in the spring. Serve it with steamed seasonal vegetables.

600g lean lamb leg meat, trimmed and cut into 3cm chunks
2 garlic cloves, finely chopped
1 tsp ground cumin
1 tsp ground coriander
½ tsp hot chilli powder
1 cinnamon stick
400g can chickpeas, rinsed and drained
400g can chopped tomatoes
2 tbsp clear honey
zest of ½ lemon
1 generous handful of fresh coriander leaves
1 small handful of toasted almonds
sea salt and freshly ground black pepper

Preheat the oven to 190°C/Gas 5. Put the meat into a casserole and add the garlic, cumin, ground coriander, chilli powder, cinnamon and chickpeas. Stir to combine. Add the tomatoes, honey and 400ml boiling water. Stir in the lemon zest, then season with a pinch of salt, if you like, and black pepper.

Cover the dish and cook in the oven for 2 hours or until the lamb is meltingly tender. Stir in the chopped coriander and sprinkle the toasted almonds on top before serving.

Beef and Mushroom Stroganoff with Tagliatelle

SERVES **4** CALS: **594** per serving

This really is a treat, for me – more of a once-a-month than a once-a-week treat, though, as it is high in calories. Keep it in your repertoire, and when the rain's pouring down, and life's feeling tough, start cooking this. Creamy, dreamy and meltingly tender – this isn't diet food, it's comfort food.

    1 small knob of butter, the size of the tip of your thumb
    1 tbsp olive oil
    400g beef rump steak, trimmed and finely sliced into
        strips 1½cm wide
    300g tagliatelle
    300g small button mushrooms, finely sliced
    2 large leeks, finely chopped
    125ml white vermouth
    400ml half-fat crème fraîche
    1 tsp Dijon mustard
    1 tsp wholegrain mustard
    chopped fresh flat-leaf parsley leaves
    sea salt and freshly ground black pepper

Bring a pan of water to the boil ready to cook the pasta. Melt half the butter and half the oil in a large, non-stick frying pan over a medium heat. Increase the heat, then quickly sear the beef in batches until browned on both sides. Remove the meat and leave to one side. Add the pasta to the pan of water and cook according to the pack instructions. Drain in a colander.

Add the remaining butter and oil to the frying pan. Add the mushrooms to the frying pan, cook to brown quickly, then leave to one side with the beef. Reduce the heat and gently fry the leeks, then return the beef and mushrooms to the pan. Add the vermouth to the frying pan and let everything bubble. Season to taste.

Put the crème fraîche in a bowl and add both mustards, then mix well together. Add this mixture to the pan and gently stir. Cook until the mixture has reduced a little then serve with the tagliatelle, with chopped parsley on top.

Beef Massaman

SERVES 4 CALS: **423** per serving without rice;
693 per serving with rice

This was one of the very first dishes on the Jane Plan menu and continues to be a favourite with Jane Plan clients.

400ml can low-fat coconut milk
4 tbsp massaman curry paste
600g beef stewing steak, cut into large chunks
450g potatoes, cut into 2.5cm chunks
1 onion, cut into thin wedges
4 fresh or frozen kaffir lime leaves
1 cinnamon stick
1 tbsp tamarind paste
1 tbsp palm sugar or soft light brown sugar
1 tbsp fish sauce
300g basmati rice
juice of 1 lime
2 red chillies, deseeded and finely sliced, to serve
1 lime, cut into wedges, to serve

Preheat the oven to 180°C/Gas 4. Heat 2 tbsp of the coconut milk in a large flameproof casserole with a lid over a medium heat. Add the curry paste and fry for 1 minute, then stir in the beef and fry until well coated and sealed. Stir in the remaining coconut milk with half a can of water, the potatoes, onion, lime leaves, cinnamon, tamarind, sugar and fish sauce. Bring to the boil, then cover and cook in the oven for 2 hours or until the beef is tender.

Twenty minutes before the end of cooking time, cook the rice in a pan of boiling water, according to the pack instructions. Remove the casserole from the oven and squeeze the lime juice into the curry, then gently stir. Scatter the sliced chilli on top and serve with the rice and lime wedges.

....

Jane Tip » *If you leave out the rice you can save 180 calories per person.*

....

Classic Chilli con Carne

SERVES **4**   CALS: **631** per serving

You may be wondering how something as innocent as the family-favourite chilli con carne made it onto the Sinner Dinner list. It's the rice – without the rice, this recipe comes in at just 349 calories, but for many people eating chilli con carne without rice is just not an option. You could, of course, combine it with Cauliflower Rice (see page 239), and make it a Thinner Dinner. I'll leave it to you. Only you know how many calories you have in your savings account. This is one of the best-sellers at Jane Plan, so here's the recipe for you to make at home.

1 tbsp sunflower oil
1 large onion, finely diced
2 garlic cloves, finely sliced
1 red pepper, deseeded and finely chopped
1 heaped tsp hot chilli powder, or to taste
500g lean minced beef
300ml beef stock (use a cube)
400g can chopped tomatoes
2 tbsp tomato purée
½ tsp dried marjoram
1 tsp sugar
400g can red kidney beans, rinsed and drained
300g basmati rice
sea salt and freshly ground black pepper

Heat the oil in a large pan over a medium heat for 1–2 minutes until hot. Add the onion and cook, stirring frequently, for 5 minutes. Add the garlic, red pepper and chilli powder. Stir well, then cook for another 5 minutes, stirring occasionally. Increase the heat to medium-high and add the minced beef. Using a spatula or wooden spoon, break up the mince as it fries and browns – make sure you keep the heat hot enough for the meat to brown rather than stew.

Pour the stock into the pan and add the tomatoes and tomato purée, marjoram and sugar. Season and stir the sauce well. Bring to the boil, then reduce the heat to low until it is gently simmering. Cook for 20 minutes. Check the pan occasionally to make sure that the sauce doesn't catch on the bottom or isn't drying out. Add 1–2 tbsp water, if needed.

Add the kidney beans and simmer for 10 minutes, adding a little more water if it looks too dry. Taste the chilli and adjust the seasoning; add extra chilli powder, if needed. Cover the pan, turn off the heat and leave the chilli to stand for 10 minutes before serving to allow the flavours to mingle. While the chilli is resting, cook the rice according to the pack instructions. Serve the chilli with the rice.

Jane Tip » *Top your chilli with low-fat crème fraîche, chopped avocado and chopped fresh chillies. This is a lovely way to jazz up a simple supper. Allow 70 extra calories per person for the avocado, assuming half an avocado each, and about 20 calories extra each for 1 tbsp crème fraîche.*

Oriental Pork with Sweet Potato and Butternut Squash

SERVES 6   CALS: 562 per serving

This makes a perfect, delicious Saturday-night supper. Once all the preparation is done, you can relax while everything gently roasts in the oven.

    2 tbsp Chinese five-spice powder
    3 tbsp olive oil
    8 tbsp soy sauce
    4 tbsp dry sherry
    2 tsp brown sugar
    1kg boneless pork loin
    1cm piece of fresh root ginger, peeled and grated
    1 tsp dried chilli flakes
    2 large sweet potatoes, peeled and cut into chunks
    3 large carrots, cut into chunks
    ½–1 medium butternut squash, peeled and cut into chunks
    sea salt

Start preparations in the morning. Put the five-spice powder in a bowl and add 1 tbsp of the olive oil, the soy sauce, sherry and sugar, and add salt to taste. Mix well and then rub the mixture all over the pork. Put the pork in the fridge to marinate during the day.

When ready to cook, preheat the oven to 200°C/Gas 6 and put the pork in a roasting tin. Roast for 1 hour.

Put the remaining olive oil in a large bowl and add the ginger and chilli flakes. Add the sweet potatoes, carrots and butternut squash, then toss to coat in the oil. When the meat has cooked for 1 hour put the vegetables in another roasting tin at the top of the oven, above the pork. Roast the pork and vegetables for 45 minutes or until the pork is cooked through.

Remove the pork from the oven, cover with foil and leave to rest for 15 minutes. Leave the vegetables to continue roasting, if needed, until golden. Serve the vegetables with the pork.

....

Jane Tip » *You can serve this for Sunday lunch and marinate the pork the night before. Being a bit of a veggie lover I like to add some green vegetables – a simple serving of steamed spinach hits the spot!*

....

TOO BUSY TO SHOP AND CHOP? GO FOR SUPERMARKET STANDBYS

Life can sometimes be such a whirl that, although you have every intention of cooking from scratch, it simply isn't possible. On those occasions, don't beat yourself up – instead, head off to the local supermarket and, if you look carefully, you'll find a range of wonderful choices that will help you stay within your calorie budget. In fact, why not be a savvy shopper and make sure you have a couple in the fridge at all times, so that when you're dog tired and can't be bothered you have something ready made, to keep you going and help you stay on track? On the following pages you'll find suggestions to get you going. Although ranges change all the time, as long as you're an avid label reader, you can't go wrong!

→

For those days when you really don't have the time to cook, supermarket ready meals can be a godsend. The following calorie-counted meals fit the Jane Plan diet guidelines. This should give you some good ideas but, as with the supermarket and sandwich shop choices for lunch, do always check the nutritional label because recipes – and, as a result, calorie counts – are often altered.

ASDA

▶ Reduced Calorie Chicken Sizzler – 275 calories

▶ Reduced Calorie Chicken in Peppercorn Sauce – 316 calories

▶ Reduced Calorie Chicken Tikka Masala & Pilau Rice – 315 calories

Marks & Spencer – Count On Us

(all main meals less than 400 calories)

▶ Count On Us Chilli Con Carne – 90 calories per 100g

▶ Count On Us Chicken in Mushroom Sauce with New Potatoes – 75 calories per 100g

▶ Count On Us Vegetable Moussaka – 70 calories per 100g

Marks & Spencer – Fuller Longer

▶ Fuller Longer Asian-style Fishcake and King Prawn noodles – 340 calories

→

- ► Fuller Longer Cod Rogan Balti with an Onion Bhajji topping – 345 calories

- ► Fuller Longer Roasted Duck and Pork Pappardelle – 340 calories

- ► Fuller Longer Beef Bourguignon with Mashed Potato and Savoy Cabbage – 315 calories

- ► Fuller Longer Keralan Chicken Curry with Spiced Samosa Crust – 320 calories

Sainsbury's – Be Good To Yourself

- ► Be Good To Yourself Prawn Biryani – 318 calories

- ► Be Good To Yourself Mediterranean Vegetable Pasta – 351 calories

- ► Be Good To Yourself Braised Beef & Mash – 311 calories

- ► Be Good To Yourself Chicken & Mushroom Pie – 349 calories

Tesco (Only 1 meal under 350 calories)

- ► Light Choices Chicken Breasts with Tomato & Basil – 154 calories per serving (half pack)

Waitrose – Love Life You Count

- ► Love Life you count Cottage Pie – 338 calories

- ► Love Life you count Chicken with Madeira wine & porcini mushrooms – 318 calories

→

▶ Love Life you count Fisherman's Pie – 285 calories

▶ Love life you count Spinach & Ricotta Cannelloni – 275 calories

EATING OUT

There's a whole section on eating out wisely pages 108–110, but here are some more ideas for when you need a treat or simply want something easy after a long hard day. Interestingly, while researching this book, very few restaurants had their calorie counts available. I feel this needs to change, as it is important, especially for those on a weight-loss journey, to be able to see at a glance the calorie count of foods on the menu. As I mentioned previously, do always check the calorie counts as recipes do change.

RESTAURANTS

Nando's

▶ Quarter Leg Peri Peri Chicken	218 calories
▶ Quarter Breast Peri Peri Chicken	135 calories
▶ Chicken Wings, three	189 calories
▶ Chicken Wings, five	296 calories
▶ Mediterranean Salad	230 calories
▶ Chicken Breast Fillet Burger	333 calories

→

Pizza Express

- Leggera Superfood Salad — 300 calories
- Pollo ad Astra Leggera Pizza (eat half) — 250 calories
- Pomodoro Pesto Leggera Pizza (eat half) — 250 calories
- Padana Leggera Pizza (eat half) — 250 calories

Yo! Sushi

- Spicy Seafood Udon — 306 calories
- Vegetable Firecracker Rice — 341 calories
- Chicken Yakisoba — 294 calories
- Prawn Yakisoba — 233 calories
- Vegetable Gyoza — 111 calories
- Chicken Gyoza — 119 calories
- Spicy Pepper Squid — 145 calories
- Prawn Tempura — 133 calories
- Tuna Sashimi — 65 calories
- Salmon Sashimi — 140 calories
- Coriander Tuna Sashimi — 75 calories
- California Hand Roll — 117 calories
- Tuna Maki — 115 calories
- Cucumber Maki — 93 calories
- Aubergine Salad — 82 calories
- Crunchy Tofu Salad — 103 calories

Chapter Eighteen

■

CALORIE CHARTS

AT JANE PLAN, we know you don't always have time for weighing and measuring, so here is a chart to help you understand how many calories there are in an average portion.

Food type	Weight	Portion size	Calories
Poultry and game			
Chicken			
Breast, skinless, grilled	125g	medium breast	170
Breast strips, stir-fried	90g	1 large handful	145
Thigh, casseroled, with skin	125g	medium thigh	130
Duck			
Roasted	185g	medium breast	361

Food type	Weight	Portion size	Calories
Turkey			
Breast, skinless, grilled	90g	small breast	140
Strips, stir fried	90g	1 large handful	148
Venison			
Roasted	120g	2 slices	198

Meat

Beef			
Braising steak, uncooked	85g	1 large handful	191
Fillet steak (sold as 100g raw) grilled	155g	medium steak	291
Mince, extra lean, stewed	140g	1 large handful	248
Rump steak (sold as 100g raw) grilled	205g	medium steak	353
Rump steak, strips, Stir-fried	103g	1 large handful	214
Sirloin steak (sold as 100g raw) grilled	155g	medium steak	272
Lamb			
Leg steaks, grilled	90g	medium steak	178
Loin chops, grilled	70g	medium chop	149
Mince, stewed	90g	1 large handful	187
Rack of lamb, roasted	90g	2 chops	203
Shoulder joint, roasted	90g	2 slices	212
Stewing, stewed	130g	1 large handful	312

→

Food type	Weight	Portion size	Cals
Pork, bacon and ham			
Rashers, back, grilled	66g	2 rashers	142
Rashers, streaky, grilled	66g	2 rashers	224
Parma ham	47g	4 slices	105
Premium ham	56g	2 slices	74
Pork shoulder, cured	100g	2 slices	103
Leg joint, roasted	90g	2 slices	164
Loin chops, grilled	75g	medium chop	140
Loin joint, pot roasted	90g	2 slices	177
Pork steaks, grilled	135g	medium steak	228
Spare rib, grilled	110g	2 ribs	321

Fish and seafood

Anchovies in oil	10g	1 anchovy	28
Cod, baked	120g	small fillet	115
Cod, poached	120g	small fillet	113
Haddock, grilled	120g	small fillet	125
Haddock, poached	120g	small fillet	136
Haddock, steamed	120g	small fillet	107
Hake, grilled	100g	small fillet	113
Halibut, grilled	145g	small fillet	175
Kipper, baked	130g	2 fillets	267
Kipper, grilled	130g	2 fillets	332
Mackerel, grilled	147g	2 fillets	351
Monkfish, grilled	70g	small fillet	67
Mussels, boiled, shelled	40g	1 handful	42
Plaice, grilled	130g	small fillet	125
Prawns, boiled, shelled	60g	1 handful	59
Salmon, grilled	82g	small fillet	176
Salmon, smoked	56g	2 slices	80

Food type	Weight	Portion size	Cals
Salmon, steamed	77g	small fillet	152
Sardines, grilled	40g	2 fillets	78
Scallops, steamed, shelled	70g	1 large handful	83
Swordfish, grilled	125g	small fillet	174
Trout, brown, grilled with skin	100g	medium fillet	98
Trout, rainbow, grilled	120g	medium fillet	162
Tuna, canned in brine	45g	1 tbsp	45
Tuna, raw	45g	2 slices	61

Rice, pasta, grains and pulses

Rice

Basmati, uncooked	75g	a tennis ball	270
White, uncooked	75g	a tennis ball	265

Pasta and grains

Bulgur wheat, cooked	84g	3 tbsp	70
Couscous, cooked	88g	3 tbsp	93
Noodles, rice, uncooked	75g	a tennis ball	147
Tagliatelle, dried, uncooked	75g	a tennis ball	262
Spaghetti, uncooked	75g	a tennis ball	270

Pulses

Butter beans, canned	118g	3 tbsp	95
Cannellini beans, canned	123g	3 tbsp	103
Chickpeas, canned	120g	3 tbsp	145
Lentils, Puy, canned	117g	3 tbsp	100
Lentils, Puy, dried and cooked (cooked weight)	125g	3 tbsp	117
Kidney beans, canned	120g	3 tbsp	125

→

Food type	Weight	Portion size	Cals
Cereals			
Bran flakes	40g	1 ramekin*	126
Cornflakes	40g	1 ramekin	144
Fruit and fibre	40g	1 ramekin	147
Muesli	40g	1 ramekin	147
Porridge, uncooked	40g	1 ramekin	148

* Ramekin size: 57 x 25mm

Food type	Weight	Portion size	Cals
Dips			
Guacamole	45g	1 tbsp	58
Hummus	30g	1 tbsp	56
Taramasalata	45g	1 tbsp	227
Tzatziki	45g	1 tbsp	30

Food type	Weight	Portion size	Cals
Cold drinks and juices			
Cola	330ml	a can	139
Apple juice	200ml	small glass	93
Diet cola	330ml	a can	trace
Grapefruit juice	200ml	small glass	82
Lemonade	200ml	small glass	36
Orange juice	200ml	small glass	87

Food type	Weight	Portion size	Cals
Coffee and tea			
Cappuccino, semi-skimmed	200ml	1 cup	63**
Coffee with semi-skimmed milk	200ml	1 cup	13
Coffee with skimmed milk	200ml	1 cup	8
Coffee with whole milk	200ml	1 cup	15
Tea, green	200ml	1 cup	trace
Tea, herbal	200ml	1 cup	2

Food type	Weight	Portion size	Cals
Tea, with semi-skimmed milk	200ml	1 cup	13
Tea, with skimmed milk	200ml	1 cup	8
Tea, with whole milk	200ml	1 cup	15

** The calories in coffee-shop cappuccinos vary greatly, partly because their servings are so huge. A 200ml serving is a small cup, the size you would probably have at home. If you buy a cappuccino or latte on the run, the chances are you'll be drinking far more calories than 63.

Cheese

Food type	Weight	Portion size	Cals
Brie	30g	1 slice	108
Camembert	30g	1 slice	87
Cheddar	30g	matchbox	124
Cottage cheese, 4% fat	40g	1 tbsp	36
Cottage cheese, 2% fat	40g	1 tbsp	28
Danish blue	30g	matchbox	103
Dolcelatte	30g	matchbox	118
Double Gloucester	30g	matchbox	123
Edam	30g	matchbox	102
Emmenthal	30g	matchbox	120
Feta	50g	1 slice	125
Gouda	30g	matchbox	113
Halloumi	40g	1 slice	124
Mozzarella	37g	¼ of a ball	87
Parmesan, freshly grated	20g	1 tbsp	82
Red Leicester	30g	matchbox	120
Ricotta	55g	1 tbsp	79
Roquefort	30g	1 slice	112
Soft light	30g	1 tbsp	47
Soft medium fat	30g	1 tbsp	74
Stilton	30g	1 slice	142

➡

Food type	Weight	Portion size	Cals
Dairy			
Milk			
Semi-skimmed	200ml	1 glass	98
Skimmed	200ml	1 glass	68
Soya sweetened	200ml	1 glass	94
Soya unsweetened	200ml	1 glass	62
Whole	200ml	1 glass	134
Cream cheese			
Crème fraîche	15ml	1 tbsp	45
Crème fraîche, low-fat	15ml	1 tbsp	25
Fromage frais, fruit	50g	small pot	55
Fromage frais, fruit, virtually fat-free	50g	small pot	23
Fromage frais, natural	100g	⅕ of a pot	46
Yoghurt			
Fat-free Greek	100g	⅕ of a large pot	57
Greek	100g	⅕ of a large pot	130
Low-fat natural	100g	⅕ of a large pot	65
Low-fat fruit	125g	small pot	100
Fruit			
Apple	160g	1 whole, medium	77
Avocado	150g	1 whole, medium	285
Banana	150g	1 whole, medium	142
Blackberries	160g	2 handfuls	42
Blueberries	160g	2 handfuls	91
Cherries	160g	2 handfuls	82
Clementine	150g	2 whole, medium	70

Food type	Weight	Portion size	Cals
Grapefruit	130g	one whole, medium	54
Grapes	160g	2 handfuls	102
Kiwi fruit	120g	2 whole, medium	50
Mango	100g	½	58
Melon	100g	1 slice	34
Nectarine	150g	1 whole, medium	54
Orange	130g	1 whole, medium	62
Peach	150g	1 whole, medium	50
Pear	160g	1 whole, medium	67
Pineapple	100g	2 slices	50
Plum	130g	2 whole, medium	60
Raspberries	160g	2 handfuls	43
Strawberries	160g	2 handfuls	45
Tangerine	140g	2 whole, medium	74

Vegetables

Food type	Weight	Portion size	Cals
Asparagus	160g	2 handfuls	32
Aubergine	160g	2 handfuls	23
Beetroot	160g	2 handfuls	46
Broccoli	160g	2 handfuls	48
Brussels sprouts	160g	2 handfuls	56
Butternut squash	160g	2 handfuls	47
Cabbage	160g	2 handfuls	34
Carrots	160g	2 handfuls	45
Cauliflower	160g	2 handfuls	50
Celery	120g	2 medium stalks	8
Courgette	160g	2 handfuls	29
Cucumber	160g	2 handfuls	16
Fennel	160g	2 handfuls	15
Green beans	160g	2 handfuls	38

→

Food type	Weight	Portion size	Cals
Iceberg lettuce	100g	2 handfuls	14
Leeks	160g	2 handfuls	35
Mangetouts	160g	2 handfuls	53
Mushrooms	160g	2 handfuls	24
Onions	160g	2 handfuls	61
Parsnips	160g	2 handfuls	99
Peas	160g	2 handfuls	116
Peppers	160g	2 handfuls	46
Spinach	100g	2 handfuls	41
Swede	160g	2 handfuls	38
Sweet potato	160g	2 handfuls	117
Sweetcorn	160g	2 handfuls	130
Tomatoes	160g	2 handfuls	28

Alcohol

Food type	Weight	Portion size	Cals
Lager	568ml	pint glass	232
Bitter	568ml	pint glass	181
Champagne	175ml	medium glass	133
Red wine	175ml	small glass	149
Red wine	250ml	large glass	212
White wine	175ml	small glass	144
White wine	250ml	large glass	205
Spirits	35ml	1 measure	81

Part Four

■

NO GOING BACK

Congratulations! You're there – you've reached your hard-earned weight-loss goal. It really is the best achievement ever, but at Jane Plan we realise that after weeks, months or even years of working towards your goal weight, the next step can be the most crucial.

Losing weight and keeping it off is easy, as long as you approach it as a long-term project. A diet will always be a quick fix if you don't take some elements of it forward to the post-weight-loss phase. A good tactic is to approach your weight in a similar way as you would, say, backache, or something you are trying to fix in your body.

For example, if you have backache and take a painkiller, the backache goes, but it returns once

→

you stop taking the painkiller; however, if while taking the painkiller, you buy a new chair, adjust your posture and start doing Pilates, you reduce the risk of your backache recurring. The reason? You have put long-term protective strategies into place.

Similarly, if you follow the Jane Plan way of eating, you will lose weight, but if once you reach your goal you simply return to your old eating habits, the weight will return. To prevent this you need to stick to the basic principles of the Skinny Rules in a balanced way, as I explain in this part of the book.

Chapter Nineteen

■

YOUR LIFE IN BALANCE

YOU MAY BE RELIEVED to know that you don't have to continue to follow the basic Skinny Rules to the letter for life. The secret is to strike a balance. On some days you can afford to eat a little more as long as on others you redress the balance by eating a little less. Alternatively, you may prefer to eat as you have been, but with a more relaxed approach. Ultimately, it's up to you to figure out a strategy that works for you; however, I am going to share with you some things I do to maintain my own weight that I know will help to keep you on the straight and narrow.

Jane Wisdom

Try sticking to the rules from Monday to Friday but take the weekend off in the early days of your post-diet phase. Alternatively, adopt a day-on/day-off approach.

REVISIT YOUR BMR

Are you happy with your new weight? If you are, now's the time to re-visit your basal metabolic rate (BMR) to help you maintain it. The reason? The lighter you are, the less energy you need each day to keep your body ticking over, which means your ideal calorie count to keep your weight stable is probably lower now than it was when you first started eating the Jane Plan way. Turn back to pages 47–8 to remind yourself how to check your BMR.

The good news is that you will no longer have to cut down your calories as you have been doing; however, this does not mean that you can just eat extra. You need to re-check your BMR to find out the ideal calorie count to maintain your current new weight. If you're nervous about adding extra calories into your day all at once, add them little by little, week by week. Keep weighing yourself, and if you find you're still losing weight, add a few more. You will soon discover exactly how much you can eat each day to stay the same weight.

Jane Wisdom

Be a calorie pessimist. Remember: whatever you fancy eating probably contains more calories than you think.

HAVE A BUFFER ZONE

Continue to weigh yourself each week and at the same time set yourself a goal weight over which you will never go. Some people find establishing a buffer zone of 2–3 pounds (900g–1.3kg) can help; for example, if your ideal weight is 9 stone 7lb (57kg), the weight over which you should never go is 9 stone 10lb (62kg). If you see your weight creeping up towards your buffer zone, you need to return to the Jane Plan Skinny Rules for at least a week. Nipping weight gain in the bud is vital, or before you know it you will be back to square one, and losing weight is much harder the second time round.

Approach your weight in the same way as your bank account. Just as the bigger your overdraft gets the more daunting and harder it becomes to clear, so it is with weight loss. Having a buffer zone will stop you going too far into the red. Some people find a good way to get round the buffer zone is to set their goal weight three pounds lighter than they actually want to be.

THINK BEFORE YOU EAT

Keeping weight off the Jane Plan way means you still need to carry on thinking before you eat, along the lines of, Is it good for me, do I need it? If you can justify it, the chances are you do and it will be OK to go ahead and eat it. But you also need to think about setting up a strategy to help redress the calorie balance; for example, if you have a cappuccino and cake during the day, go for a simple salad or soup for supper.

Jane Wisdom
Be eternally vigilant – it's the only way to keep weight off for good.

BE DRINK AWARE

Cutting back on alcohol remains one of the hardest challenges during and post weight loss. At Jane Plan, while we really do know what a difference that 'wine o'clock' moment can make to stressful lives, we also know how dangerous it can be to celebrate your weight loss by re-introducing the drinking hour. To make it easier, try allowing yourself wine two nights a week or, if that is still too hard to bear, every other night. But remember: never have more than two glasses.

By now, hopefully, you will have dropped your cappuccino or latte habit and become a herbal tea lover. But what if you can't do without that cup of coffee for a day longer? Make it a once-a-week treat. Saturday morning, for example, is a wonderful time to linger over a cappuccino.

KEEP DRINKING WATER

Water really is your best friend – staying hydrated will make you feel more energised and less hungry. This is an easy habit to keep going and one that not only makes you feel better but it will also make you look better. Benefits include clear skin, sparkly eyes and silky hair. Remember: as a Jane Planner you are now a water devotee for life.

NEVER, NEVER NIBBLE

As you know only too well, losing weight the Jane Plan way has a strict no-nibbling policy, and this is the one rule you can't afford to break – ever. You need to stick to the Jane Plan principle of three meals a day with two snacks in between.

Carry on looking at the healthy Jane Plan snack list on pages 146–8 for inspiration for 80 per cent of the time and introduce a scone or cake as a weekend treat. A treat is only a treat if you have it occasionally. If you have your treat every day it quickly becomes a habit.

Jane Wisdom
Don't get side-tracked. Every calorie still counts. Practise portion control.

By now you will have got used to eating significantly smaller portions, but you do need to take care they don't creep up in size. You can, however, afford to add a few extras such as an extra roast potato at Sunday lunch, the occasional poppadom with a curry or a plate of pasta.

To keep my weight under control I have little rules that I follow, like no more than two potatoes with Sunday lunch, and a maximum of one takeaway a month. Think about your potential 'weaknesses' and make your own list of little rules.

Jane Wisdom
You still need to be able to see the porcelain on your plate at every meal.

CONTINUE YOUR CARB CURFEW

Now you have reached your weight-loss goal you can relax the carb curfew; however, many people find that they have so enjoyed eating more vegetables at supper that they can do without the carbs for good. It's up to you to decide.

If you relax the carb curfew, make sure you keep an eye on portion control and remember the rules – your rice or pasta portion should be about the size of a tennis ball, and potatoes should be around the size of a small computer mouse.

Jane Wisdom
If you've had a big night out, balance it by watching your calories carefully the following day.

KEEP ON THE MOVE

As I explained in Skinny Rule 8, exercise is the cornerstone of weight maintenance, not only because moving uses calories but also because of the beneficial effect it has on overall health and well-being. I hope that now you have learned to love the fact that you are moving more, so it's time to step up the tempo by increasing the type of exercise you do each day.

What kind of mover are you? Take a look at the chart opposite.

Jane Wisdom
Throw away your fat clothes – you won't need them again.

WHAT KIND OF MOVER ARE YOU?

You are a ...	Your lifestyle	Aim to ...
Slow mover	Desk job. Sedentary. Tapping feet under desk, getting up to talk rather than emailing	Park the car a little further away from home and work. Plan a decent walk every weekend. Think about doing a sponsored walk
Medium mover	Sedentary but probably walking rather than taking public transport. Exercising at least once a week	Sign up for a weekly class at the gym. Increase the pace of your weekend walk to a jog. Consider signing up for an event – like a 3k run
Mean mover	Active. Regular gym-goer	Increase the intensity of your current activities. Put some variety into your routine, such as run three times a week, add a yoga or Pilates class, or some resistance training. Put your name down for a 5k, 10k, half-marathon or even a marathon

Chapter Twenty

■

THE JANE PLAN LIFESTYLE

NOW YOU HAVE REACHED the post-diet stage it is time to start enjoying every aspect of the wonderful new you. And as long as you remember the basic Jane Plan Skinny Rules, which by now will have become second nature, the good news is that there is no reason why you cannot stay super-slim.

Life after Jane Plan is not just about counting calories, though. There are other factors to consider, such as a good sleep routine, keeping stress to a minimum and being body aware. These can all help you make the most of your new lifestyle and put you in a better place to maintain the fabulous new shape you have worked so hard to achieve.

AIM TO SLEEP BETTER

What's sleep got to with weight control? If you don't get enough sleep, research shows that your body will crave high-fat foods and sweets and will trigger overeating to keep you going. A study from the New York Obesity Research Centre at St Luke's Roosevelt Hospital throws some intriguing light on this.

The researchers discovered that sleep deprivation actually altered the brain circuitry so that unhealthy foods seemed more attractive. The people they studied ate more often and went for fattier foods as well as consuming around 300 more calories on the day they were sleep deprived. And we all know where such eating habits lead: to a disappointing result on weigh-in day.

That's not all. It is also thought that if you don't get enough sleep your metabolism slows down to conserve energy. This triggers the release of the stress hormone cortisol, which is thought to increase hunger. The body thinks it needs more energy, so it asks for food. At the same time, lack of sleep also interferes with the control of two other hormones, ghrelin – aka the 'hunger hormone' that increases appetite, especially for high-carb foods – and leptin, the hormone that tells your stomach that it is full and to stop eating. The result? A galloping – and unstoppable – appetite for unhealthy foods.

Night-time soothers

For optimal health, most experts suggest you get about eight hours' sleep a night. If you are clocking up less than this, here are some tips to help yourself to a better night.

▶ **Get into a sleep routine** Go to bed and wake up at the same time each day – even on the weekends.

▶ **Be a nifty napper** A nap can boost brainpower, but if they are taken after 3.00pm a nap might make it harder for you to fall asleep at night.

▶ **Sleep-proof your bedroom** Get rid of anything that might distract you from sleep, such as noises, bright lights, an uncomfortable bed, or a TV or computer. Your bedroom is for sleep and sex only.

▶ **Relax, relax** Take time to unwind before going to bed. Make a relaxing activity, such as reading or listening to soothing music, part of your bedtime ritual.

▶ **Take up evening yoga classes** Yoga, Pilates and other stretching techniques done late in the day can help relax muscles and may help to beat insomnia.

▶ **Resist late-night viewing** Turn off the TV an hour before you go to bed to allow your brain to settle.

▶ **Eat wisely** Avoid large meals, caffeine, alcohol and nicotine close to bedtime.

▶ **Do something different** If you can't get to sleep, don't just lie there tossing and turning. Get up, go to the next-door room and read a book, do a crossword or a jigsaw.

STRESS CAN MAKE YOU FAT

We all need some stress in our lives, but too much can be harmful, especially to your waistline. We all know how easy it is to reach for the biscuit tin when under pressure, be it from screaming children, constant work demands or just the ups and downs of everyday living. Sometimes the stressful moment passes, but if you stay stressed out for a prolonged amount of time your health can be at risk.

The reason? Stress triggers the 'fight or flight response', a primitive reaction that helped our Stone Age ancestors deal with danger. Your body reacts to stress as if it is in danger and starts to release stress hormones, including cortisol, which as well as getting the body ready for action slows down metabolism and triggers cravings for fatty, sugary foods to keep you going. If the stress is a one-off situation this doesn't matter much, as your body burns off the extra calories. But chronic stress that goes on day in and day out, causing you to eat like this all the time, inevitably leads to weight gain.

What's more, it is now known that high cortisol levels lead to the body laying down fat in the abdominal area and around the vital organs rather than storing it on the hips. This fat around the middle has become known as 'toxic fat' as it produces inflammatory chemicals that are linked with an increased risk of type-2 diabetes, heart disease and stroke.

How to bust stress

▶ **Stay active** Regular exercise – 30 minutes most days – triggers the release of the body's happy hormone, serotonin, and helps dissipate cortisol. Brisk walking, dancing and swimming are all good options.

▶ **Get your work–life balance right** Overwork is a common stress trigger. Part-time or flexible working, or working from home, may be an answer.

▶ **De-clutter** Living surrounded by piles of clutter can be very stressful, especially when you can't find the necessities of life, like the front-door keys. Aim to tidy one room a week and then keep it that way.

▶ **Relax** Chilling out can reduce stress and keep you calm. Soak in a warm bath, take a walk in the park, or watch an uplifting film.

▶ **Eat right** Put calming foods on the menu, such as oats, turkey and cottage cheese, and drink plenty of soothing herbal teas, such as camomile and valerian. If you can, avoid alcohol. It may relax you in the short term, but the chances are the after effects will make things worse.

▶ **Have a giggle** Laughter is the best medicine. Nothing seems quite so stressful if you can laugh about it.

▶ **Take time out** Go for a walk in the sunshine, sign up for a yoga class, go window-shopping – the important thing is to enjoy yourself.

▶ **Plan ahead** Avoid overflowing in-trays, missed deadlines and unfulfilled commitments by not saying yes to everyone and everything. Instead, delegate wherever possible and map out your time well in advance.

TAKE A DEEP BREATH

Try this quick and simple exercise if you start to feel stressed. Keep your breathing smooth and regular throughout.

1. Sit or lie in a comfortable position with your arms and legs uncrossed and your spine straight.

2. Breathing from your abdomen, inhale through your nose, slowly to a count of five.

3. Pause and hold your breath for a count of five.

4. Exhale through your mouth or nose to a count of five.

5. When you have exhaled completely, take two breaths in your normal rhythm, then repeat steps 2 to 4.

6. Repeat the exercise for at least 3 minutes.

BE A CONFIDENT BUNNY

Now that you are happy and pleased with your new shape, it's important that you stay that way, and feeling confident about how good you look will help you to do just that. Confidence builds confidence, especially when it comes to your body, but you may have to work at it. Don't worry, though, it doesn't require a lot of effort – and, best of all, it will be worth it. The reason? The better you feel about yourself the more likely you are to stick to your weight-loss plans. But what if low self-esteem thoughts start to plague your mind? The answer is to put self-doubt to rest and focus on the good things about yourself instead.

Jane Wisdom
Feeling confident about yourself will help you forget about the biscuit tin.

Feel-good tips

▶ **Be positive** If you start to think negative thoughts about your body, write down all the positive attributes and how better life is with your new weight.

▶ **Select your friends** Spend time with people who appreciate the new-look you and are supportive of your efforts to maintain your weight loss and live a healthier life.

▶ **Mirror it** Don't avoid looking at your body in mirrors or windows. Appreciate the reflection you see – it is a way to measure your success.

▶ **Stop comparing** Wishing you had someone else's long legs or flat bum just detracts from your uniqueness. Making the most of what you have got will minimise the things you don't like.

▶ **Dress up** Get rid of all those 'fat' clothes and celebrate the new you with a new dress, scarf and jewellery. It will brighten up your image and make you feel so good about yourself.

Jane Wisdom
Wear a tight-fitting dress and hopefully the thought of the slightest bulge will be enough to discourage you from mindless 'picking'.

▶ **Get frisky** Around 85 per cent of women report that having sex makes them feel good about their shape – and you will be burning off calories too.

▶ **Spoil yourself** Have a long, warm, soothing bath, massage yourself with a delicious-smelling aromatherapy oil, read an inspiring book or simply set time aside to just sit and be. After all, you deserve it.

Jane Wisdom
If you do find the pounds are creeping back, belt up one notch tighter as a reminder not to overindulge.

Chapter Twenty One

∎

HIGH DAYS AND HOLIDAYS

THERE ARE KEY POINTS in the year, such as Christmas and holidays, of which you need to be aware, when your weight will inevitably increase. But there is no need to beat yourself up about putting on weight during these periods – life and food are there to be enjoyed. Celebrations invariably involve food, and you would have to be a saint not to gain a few pounds while enjoying them. I am sure even the skinniest super-model stands on the scales on 3 January and is filled with dismay.

IT'S A BALANCING ACT!

Remember to treat your weight in the same way as you would your bank balance: sometimes it goes up, sometimes it goes down. You can adopt two strategies to deal with holiday or Christmas weight gain: a savings strategy or a repayment strategy. If you opt for a savings strategy you need to have some spare calories in the bank *before* your holiday or Christmas. That means being super-careful in the run up to these events and getting your weight a little lower than it usually is, so that you can eat (or spend) freely on Christmas Day or when relaxing on holiday. The net result is that you do gain a few pounds, but ultimately you end up at your ideal weight.

If you opt for a repayment strategy, it works the other way round. Post-Christmas or summer holidays, get back on the scales with determination. You will probably have a calorie 'overdraft' – in other words, you will have put on weight and now it's payback time. You need to spend the next few weeks carefully following the Skinny Rules. Do this and your holiday weight will be gone in no time at all.

The best strategy when it comes to high days and holidays is to adopt a damage-limitation strategy. That way, you may gain a few pounds, but if it's only a few, they are easy to deal with. When it comes to holiday weight, it's a case of easy come, easy go – as long as you deal with it the Jane Plan way!

CHRISTMAS CALORIES

Statistics show the average weight gain over Christmas is around 7 pounds (3.17kg). Of course, it is the one time of year you must be able to indulge, but no one wants to spend the whole of January trying to lose those unwanted pounds. The good news is that if you celebrate Christmas the Jane Plan way, you may put on a few pounds but it will certainly be no more than two to three. Here's how to stand up to the festive food fest and still have fun.

> *Jane Wisdom*
> The average woman has to walk four miles to cancel out the calories of a single Christmas treat. One mince pie can clock up as many as 360 calories.

The lead-up

Remember that Christmas is more than just one day – in fact most of the damage to our waistlines happens before 25 December. Here's how to manage your party season, the Jane Plan way:

▶ If you are invited to more than two parties a week, pick the one you really want to go to and enjoy yourself while being a little more restrained at the others. That way you conserve your energy for the next do and can still get into your little black dress.

▶ Agree to be the designated driver. You'll earn some brownie points, save money on cabs and drink a lot less.

▶ Remember the 'three canapés is enough' rule.

▶ Drink plenty of water!

▶ Focus on your friends rather than the food.

▶ If you sit down to eat, remember the 'eat a third less' Jane Plan principle.

▶ Keep the 'No Naughty Nibbling' rule in your head at all times. That way you can sit down to dinner knowing that you haven't blown your calorie count before you even get to the table.

▶ Bowls of chocolates, nuts, crisps and dates can add an extra 1,000 calories a day without you even noticing, so steer clear.

Jane Wisdom

We all know that nuts are healthy, but do be careful, as they can be very high in calories. Check our Skinny Snacks list in Chapter 16 to see how many calories there are in nuts, and think twice before grabbing a handful at a drinks party.

Get waisted

Most Christmas celebrations are centred on alcohol, so how can you have fun without ruining your waistline?

▶ Have three sips of water for every sip of wine.

▶ Stick to champagne – it's lower in calories than wine.

▶ Say no to after-dinner liqueurs. Not only are they are full of sugar but they will also give you the most terrible hangover.

▶ Buy the best wine you can afford – and savour every sip. If you are currently drinking a bottle of cheaper wine a night with your partner, work out how much you are spending a week and spend the equivalent on one expensive bottle, but make it last the week. You'll appreciate it much more, drink it more slowly and, as a result, cut the overall amount you drink. Remember: on Jane Plan it's all about quality not quantity. And you can certainly justify it at this time of the year!

On the big day – Christmas lunch

▶ Choose lean white turkey meat, and remove the skin. Have just one chipolata, one bacon roll, one roast potato and one tablespoon of bread sauce. Pile your plate high with veggies. That way everyone sees you have a full plate, but it will be a full plate loaded with lower calories options – and you still get to taste all the Christmas treats.

▶ Mince pies are delicious but loaded with calories – so make sure there are some clementines to have instead.

▶ Have a tablespoonful of Christmas pudding with yoghurt or crème fraîche, rather than brandy butter or cream. If you must have brandy butter, one dessertspoon is quite enough.

▶ Say no to the Christmas chocolates and start on the washing-up instead – it will stop you nibbling and earn you more brownie points. If you have to lie – then lie! 'Chocolates give me a headache.'

▶ Go for a good, long walk in the afternoon.

▶ If someone mentions supper, jump up and offer to help prepare it. Make sure to include some salad. Turkey sandwiches are loaded with calories, but a light salad will show that you are joining in and eating.

▶ Have fun, relax and remember that a little of what you fancy won't harm you.

Boxing Day bliss

Make a fabulous green salad to go with the Christmas lunch leftovers and pile your plate high with the leaves rather than cold roast potatoes. Everything must be gone by 6.00pm. If not, you have four choices – invite the neighbours round, give it to charity, freeze it or bin it.

Jane Wisdom
By 27 December the remnants of Christmas lunch should be gone for ever, or you risk grazing until the end of the year.

HOLIDAYS

Holidays provide the perfect opportunity to introduce new habits and break any old ones that may have crept in. Take advantage of new tastes and smells and try out new dishes inspired by ethnic influences, but remember that if you are not careful, delicious local food and wine can soon pile back the pounds.

Hot holidays

Enjoy the local cuisine and focus on the fresh fruit and vegetables – keep an eye out for varieties not available in the UK. Stay hydrated throughout the day, but don't be tempted by exotic juices. Keep your trusty water bottle to hand instead.

For breakfast Avoid pastries, bread and croissants. If temptation becomes too much, make one morning a week your special treat morning and have a croissant, a waffle, a pancake, some baklava or whatever the regional speciality is. The rest of the time, feast on the local fruit and add yoghurt for a beautiful Mediterranean or tropical breakfast.

For lunch Go for salads or grilled fish with fresh vegetables, and avoid the bread basket. It can be hard to resist picking over long lunches around a table filled with family or friends, so decide what you are going to eat before you sit down, and soak up the atmosphere, rather than the food. Try to have wine-free lunches – save this treat for the evenings!

For dinner Whether cooking in your villa, eating in a restaurant or having a buffet in a hotel, portion control is always your best friend. Savour the delicious local food, but make sure you can see the porcelain on your plate.

Jane Wisdom
French baguettes may be very good, but remember they are loaded with calories and readily available in the UK – save your calories for other treats.

HOLIDAY TIPS FOR THE SLIM YOU

▶ In Italy, make pasta or pizza a once-a-week treat, however much you like it.

▶ In Greece, avoid the heavy regional dishes such as moussaka, which are often laden with fat. Go for a Greek salad, grilled fish or souvlaki instead.

▶ In France, enjoy a great steak, with lots of salad, but no French fries – and no bread.

→

> ▶ In Spain, watch out for the tapas. Although they may be just a mouthful, six pieces make a good dinner.
>
> ▶ In the Caribbean, avoid those exotic fruit cocktails.
>
> ▶ In Asia, if eating curry, apply the 'rice' rule: stick to a tennis-ball-sized portion.
>
> ▶ In the USA or Australia, the 'eat one-third less' rule doesn't apply – it's eat *50 per cent less* in these countries to keep control of portions.

Jane Wisdom

Make time to swim. Thirty minutes of breaststroke will burn 367 calories, so a few gentle lengths in the pool can help you burn off the excess from the night before.

Cold holidays

If you're lucky enough to go on a skiing holiday you've probably found that it's almost impossible not to gain weight – the food is delicious, but the portions are huge and the ingredients usually rich. Although skiing may provide the perfect opportunity to move more, don't be fooled – unless you are of Olympic standard or a complete beginner using energy constantly falling over and getting up, it does not burn as many calories as you might think. Most skiers end up consuming far more calories than they are expending.

For breakfast A bowl of porridge will keep you going for longer as well as giving you more energy to perform well on the piste.

Mid morning A glass of water rather than a cappuccino will help fend off dehydration and help you ski better.

For lunch Portions tend to be huge in mountain restaurants, so share a dish with your partner or children – especially if you choose a pasta-based dish. As every skier knows, these are enormous. Go for local soups instead. Try to manage without a glass of Glühwein at lunch.

Mid afternoon Sip a cup of warming tea, but say no to Alpine pastries and cakes.

For dinner If you have succumbed to a carb-heavy lunch, stick to a simple dinner, which includes plenty of protein and lots of vegetables. Avoid heavy cheese sauces and practise portion control at all times.

Jane Wisdom
Dip crudités, rather than bread, into the fondue and try to stick to just one fondue a week.

INDEX